NO BULL BEAUTY
Cutting Through the Crap

A No-Nonsense Guide to Holistic Beauty and Wellness

For book orders, comments, product inquiries, or to schedule a consultation, email info@nobullbeauty.com.

The author has performed research to provide correctness but assumes no responsibility for errors, inaccuracies, omissions, or any inconsistencies herein.

All statements made about specific products, foods, or lifestyle choices have not been evaluated by the United States Food and Drug Administration (FDA) and are not intended to diagnose, treat, cure, or prevent disease.

All information provided in this book, or any information contained on the corresponding website is for informational purposes only and is not intended to diagnose or treat any medical condition. Always consult with a qualified healthcare professional before starting any new vitamin, supplement, or skin care regimen, diet, or exercise program. Consult a physician before taking any medication or product recommended herein, or before starting a diet. If you have a health problem, including acute or chronic disease and/or a skin condition, please seek attention from a qualified professional.

ISBN-10: 1482799200
ISBN-13: 978-1482799200

Manufactured in the United States of America

www.NoBullBeauty.com

ACKNOWLEDGMENTS

This holistic beauty guide could not have happened without the people who helped me move through life's obstacles and stood by my side every step of the way.

I would like to thank my mom, Rita. She suffered through all of my food allergies, skin sensitivities, sneezing and, of course, a few (ha!) mood swings throughout my childhood.

At a very young age, my pediatrician advised my mom to eliminate all artificial flavorings, colorings, and preservatives (BHA, BHT) from my diet. Keep in mind, I grew up when all things chemical and artificial were considered "ok" and were found in practically every product on every store shelf. My poor mom! While most kids were reading Dr. Seuss, I was reading food labels and learning how to pronounce crappy chemical names. I love you and thank you for being such a caring and loving crap-crusader mama.

I also owe gratitude to my late maternal grandmother, Josephine. Granny Jo was from Italy and accustomed to growing and using herbs and natural remedies for healing. Her wisdom and knowledge of plants inspired me and taught me valuable lessons that I use every day of my life.

Huge hugs to all the amazing family, friends, mentors, clients, Mother Nature (my other mama), and all who continuously encourage me. I love you all.

And a very special thanks to the incredible ladies that assisted me with this project and/or encouraged me along the way: Kara, Roxanne, Lisa, Leslie, Brittany, Connie, and Sarah. I am so grateful for your assistance, feedback, encouragement, support, and friendship. I am blessed to have you in my life. Thank you!

And of course, I must thank my beautiful husband, Jeff. Thank you, thank you, thank you for the endless washing of your hands and face with only the finest, most pure natural ingredients so I can be touched and kissed without breaking out in hives!

I LOVE you and thank you for being a part of my No Bull life.

Dedication

Stephen, not a day goes by that I don't think of you and miss your smile and laughter. You "got me" and my differences when nobody else did. You gave meaning to the words "brotherly love." Our Earth sign similarities and love for all things nature, pets, planet, and the great outdoors have continually inspired me to make a difference. Thank you for teaching me that it's OK to be me, to be different, to goof off, and to take chances.

I dedicate this book to you for your unconditional love and endless support. I Love You.

'Til We Meet Again,
Sher

MY JOURNEY

You may wonder what inspired me to pursue a career in Aesthetics. It's simple: I grew up battling allergies to processed foods and common ingredients found in modern body care creams, lotions, and cosmetics.

Unfortunately, I could not indulge in the drugstore options like other teens because of my severe and often painful reactions. My Italian grandmother used plant-based remedies that actually worked, which guided me to an ancestrally inspired career in aesthetics.

For the past 25 years, I have practiced as a Holistic Aesthetician customizing botanical skin treatments for a myriad of grateful clients. My studies of Holistic Wellness, Anti-Aging, Nutrition, Aromatherapy, Ayurveda, and Cosmetic Chemistry have led me down the No Bull path, enabling me to provide clients with non-toxic treatment options while I also pursue animal and planet advocacy - my other heartfelt passion. Currently a product formulator and owner of a private skin care studio, I continue to educate professionals, provide client services, and consult with other manufacturers.

My mission is to share what I have learned and experienced with anyone who is interested in knowing how to naturally nurture their health and beauty. Use this book as a reference to eliminate all the crap from your home, beauty regimen, and diet – not just for a more vibrant you but also for a happier, crap-free planet.

CONTENTS

PREFACE   xv

INTRODUCTION
Chemicals: A Brief History   17

CHAPTER 1
Does Your Beauty Routine STINK?

Conduct a No Bull Beauty Raid   22
'Sup with Sulfates?   25
The Three Pesky Ps   27
Dimethicone and Other Sneaky Silicones   30
Fragrances, Formaldehyde, and Other Funky Crap   33
Hydroquinone Belongs Down the Throne!   35
Beware of Benzoyl Peroxide   36
Last Call for Alcohol?   37
Tricky Triclosan   40
The Skinny on Sunscreen   40
Are Sunless Tans Really Worth It?   46
Poisonous Polish? P.U.!   48
Pore-Clogging Crap   49
Does Your Deodorant Stink?   51
Heavy Metal Makeup Doesn't Rock!   54
Mineral Makeup Madness   56
Funky-Fresh Preservatives   58

CHAPTER 2
The Lowdown on Labels

Confusing Label Lingo   60
Bogus Beauty Claims   61
Stinky INCI Names   64
Confused by Cosmeceuticals?   66
Don't Panic Over Organic   67
Say No to GMOs!   69

CHAPTER 3
The Scoop on Your Skin

Getting to Know the Skin You're In   73
The Differing Decades of Aging   76
Annoying Acne   79
Wicked Rosacea and Redness Relief   84
Dreaded Dark Circles and Aging Eyes   87
Awful Age Spots and Pigment Problems   89
You Can't Win with Dry Skin   91
The Fight Against Free Radicals   93
Inflammation Nation   95

CHAPTER 4
Beauty Gone Wild

Fillers, Drillers and Lasers OH MY!   97
Botox®: Miracle or Mirage?   100
Do Scrubs + Scrapers = Time Erasers?   102
Why Toy with Retinoids?   107

Hair Loss Hazards   110
Lash and Brow Lowdown   113
Luscious Lip Tips   115

CHAPTER 5
Crap-Free Living and Lifestyle

Multi-Purpose Cabinet Keepers   117
Ayurveda- Ancient Medicine for No Bull Beauty   132
Essential Oil Essentials   135
Are You Loyal to Oil?   140
Foods to Flush   142
Viva La Veggies   146
Cuckoo for Coconuts?   150
Super Duper Beauty Boosters   152
Beauty Supplements and Superfood Sources   158
To D or Not to D   168
Somethin' Fishy 'Bout Fish Oil   171
Mind/Body Beauty   173
Yoga for Youth   177
No Bull -- Get Your Beauty Sleep!   181

Finale: Top Ten No Bull Beauty Tips!

Healthy Holistic Habits   185

ABOUT THE AUTHOR   190
REFERENCES   192

PREFACE

This No Bull Beauty Guide is based on more than 25 years of meticulous research and experience as a holistic beauty expert and advocate for safe cosmetics, beauty products, and non-toxic living. My goal is simple: to help you make safer choices for yourself, your family, and even your pets. And of course, to help you achieve natural beauty!

Having always been prone to redness, breakouts and inflammation, which often led to scarring, I needed an alternative to the over-the-counter remedies, which only exacerbated my challenges. Thanks to my training and experience, I have been able to resolve my own super-sensitive skin challenges. Helping others then became my primary focus.

Unfortunately, over the past decade alone I have observed an overwhelming increase in the occurrence of common skin sensitivities ranging from redness, adult acne, and inflammatory conditions such as rosacea, as well as intolerance to many skincare ingredients. The cause of this is clearly a result of both environmental factors and toxic and irritating ingredients found in so many beauty products. In this book, you will learn when to flush beauty products and run, what those confusing labels really mean, how to determine what's crap and what's not, and how you can improve your health, appearance and the environment by making better choices in your daily routine. Most consumers are unaware that some of the most commonly used skincare ingredients are also considered allergens and are responsible for chronic skin problems as well. The loose standards for labeling of "natural" products are misleading.

So what's the answer to all of the Bull$h!t out there? Self-education is the key. In this Beauty Guide, I will teach you how to get to know yourself, your skin and your ingredients – *No Bull!*

It's now time for you to start learning and begin living a non-toxic No Bull Beauty Lifestyle. Enjoy!

INTRODUCTION

Chemicals: A Brief History

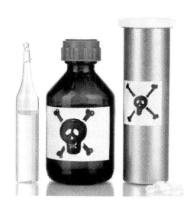

Over time, words that are overused or misused can sometimes lose their true meanings in society, especially in the modern age of electronic media and TV commercials, with the constant bombardment of advertising containing powerful ideas and subliminal messages. A good example of a word whose meaning has been altered in our minds is: chemicals.

We've come to think that all chemicals are bad. However, what many people may not realize is the simple scientific fact that without chemicals, there would be no life! Everything we see in the world, every feeling we feel, every function of our bodies, as well as those of plant life, is made possible by chemical reactions. The key, however, is distinguishing the good from the bad, which up until today has been a difficult task. In the meantime, it is up to every individual to take charge and eliminate as many negative elements from their life as possible.

It is the man-made (synthetic) chemicals and their overuse that pose the real threat. Numerous food and personal care manufacturers use the term "chemical-free" to promote their products. However, these marketing terms do not necessarily mean that these products do not contain chemicals. It is the synthetic chemicals they are referring to. Unfortunately, with no strict criteria for such claims such as "natural," "chemical-free," or "additive-free," harmful man-made chemicals may be present. The average consumer is unaware that toxic mass-produced chemicals are now the source of numerous health and environmental issues. The key is getting to know your ingredients and any potential hazards associated with them, and not to be blindsided by bogus claims.

Beginning in the 20th century, manufacturers of foods, makeup, personal care, and cleaning products found it was cheaper and more lucrative for them to create chemicals rather than use natural substances derived from the planet. The birth of processed foods was the beginning of a longer shelf life and foods that retained their freshness far beyond what had been previously thought possible. Cosmetics cost less to manufacture because they didn't require mining of natural resources like minerals and so forth, and synthetic drugs were easier to produce than natural medicinal plants which require land, time to harvest, and have a limited time span for usability. While some things may be necessary, some ingredients pose more harm than others.

The man-made chemicals that make up so much of our modern world were initially viewed as one of the best advancements in the history of humankind until the consequences of veering from nature became evident. The allergies, cancers, pollution, animal testing, factory farming, pesticides, hazardous wastes, and the long list of negative side effects from exposure to these toxic enemies are now documented and confirmed.

It's important to remember, though, that all chemicals are *not* bad and that they make up our bodies, our planet, and give us the ability to live and breathe. Chemicals are everywhere and in everything. It is many of the synthetic chemicals that are proven to be toxic and negatively impact our lives with illness, death, and the destruction of our beautiful planet. So ask yourself, "How can I avoid the toxic, synthetic, chemical crap?" Truth be known, they are everywhere in our environment. My goal is simple: to arm you with the information you need to enable yourself to distinguish between nature's chemicals and the toxic, synthetic "chemical crap." Of course, you will choose when, how, and whether or not to apply that information.

1

Does Your Beauty Routine STINK?

The skin is your body's largest organ, so a good rule of thumb is to always USE CAUTION before applying anything to your precious body without first knowing what the product contains. Studies have shown that a high percentage of chemical substances applied to the skin can end up invading your body and enter the bloodstream. Furthermore, it is estimated that at least 146 cosmetic ingredients contain carcinogenic (cancer-causing) contaminants. A 2004 study by a non-profit organization called The Environmental Working Group found that 80 percent of all cosmetic products may be contaminated with one or more carcinogenic impurities including: 1,4-dioxane, hydroquinone, ethylene dioxide, formaldehyde, nitrosamines, polyaromatic hydrocarbons, and acrylamides.[1]

Since what you put on your skin is likely to travel throughout your entire body, you must be careful of some of the toxic products on the market. There is a long list of icky ingredients that can cause inflammation (which leads to aging) and may also contribute to chronic health problems and more. However, this No Bull Beauty Guide can help you say goodbye to the confusion and headache of trying to decipher ingredient labels and figuring out what is safe to use. It's time to cut through the crap and get serious about your beauty regimen!

Your skin acts as the first line of defense against harmful invaders, much in the same way that the Earth's atmosphere protects the planet. Sneaky substances should not invade our bodies or our beautiful planet, but unfortunately it is mostly our own actions that weaken these defense systems.

Luckily, there are non-toxic ingredients and alternatives to the toxic chemical invaders of our precious bodies and our ecosystem, but there are also imposters that pose as safe products that are really total bull. So, let's get started on getting you the information you'll need to be a smart, savvy, and suspicious consumer!

Conduct a No Bull Beauty Raid

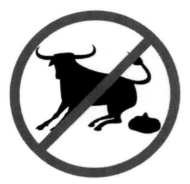

Before adding a toxic beauty product to your collection and putting another potentially harmful ingredient onto and into your body, go ahead and raid your cupboards, purse, drawers, cabinets, closets, between the mattresses, whatever!

Presently, there are more than 100 synthetic ingredients directly linked to cancer, endocrine disorders, and birth defects. The key to being truly beautiful lies within you. Make smarter choices for your body and the environment, and help change the fate of future generations by avoiding the negative consequences associated with synthetic, chemical-laden beauty products.

Ban the Top 15 Toxic Ingredients

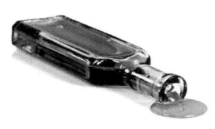

It's hard to tell just by reading the label whether an ingredient is safe. Even if it's hard to spell, read, or understand, it may not actually be bad for you. There is a lot of confusing stuff out there! Did you know as much as 78 percent of the chemicals in the highest volume of commercial use have not even undergone minimal toxicity testing?[2] Yikes!

It's no joke. According to the EPA (Environmental Protection Agency), there are currently more than 80,000 chemicals listed or registered for use, many of which have not been thoroughly assessed for their potential health and environmental risks.[3]

Check out the top 15 toxic invaders, and get ready to toss them!

1. **Aluminum:** Toxic metal found in antiperspirants, linked to Alzheimer's disease and respiratory and neurological disorders.[15]

2. **Ammonia:** Irritating to your skin, scalp, eyes, and even lungs. Found in permanent hair color. *Scary stuff.*

3. **FD&C Color and Pigments:** Heavy metals (including lead) present from coal tar that contribute to skin sensitivity and irritation, along with serious health risks.

4. **DEA, MEA & TEA (Diethanolamine, Triethanolamine and Monethanolamine):** Highly toxic and carcinogenic compounds used to form *1,4 Dioxane*. Irritating to the skin and eyes.

5. **Dimethicone and Silicones:** Non-biodegradable, clogs pores, and may contribute to premature aging.

6. **DMDM Hydantoin & Urea:** Cosmetic preservatives that release formaldehyde. May cause skin irritation, allergies, joint pain and possibly even cancer.

7. **GMOs:** Genetically modified organisms that are manipulated in a way that may pose harm to our health and the environment.

8. **Hexane, Acetone (good ol' nail polish remover) and Methanol:** Toxic chemical solvents and also a known neurotoxin and pulmonary irritant.

9. **Parabens:** Concentrations of parabens have been found in scientific studies within human breast tumors and are thought to contribute to tumorigenesis.[4]

10. **PPD - P-Phenylenediamine:** Common chemical in hair dye; toxic to the immune system, skin, nervous system and respiratory system.

11. **Petroleum Distillates (Petrochemicals):** Synthetic emollients linked to the creation of hormone inhibitors and harmful, unstable molecules known as free radicals.

12. **Hydroquinone:** Skin lightener; toxic to lungs, the nervous system, and mucous membranes. Hazardous to eyes, skin and a potential carcinogen.

13. **Phthalates and Synthetic Fragrances:** Toxic substances, dangerous when inhaled or applied topically. Non-biodegradable and known hormone disruptors.
14. **Sulfates:** Highly allergenic and irritating to the eyes and skin. Commonly used foaming agents.
15. **Triclosan:** Antibacterial agent suspected of causing cancer in humans.

Selecting products without some of these commonly used bad boys and other synthetic ingredients is the first step to greening your beauty routine!

Now, let's review some of them a bit more in detail.

'Sup with Sulfates?

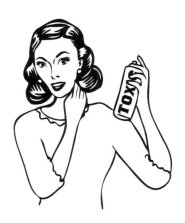

You have likely seen commercials promoting "sulfate-free" products, which indicates that we are finally speaking loud enough to bring about positive change. However, you need to read labels because many manufacturers are still using sulfates in their products. Here is a rundown on sulfates and why you should avoid them.

Sulfates are grease-cutting chemicals that act as foaming agents when used in shampoos and/or cleansers. There are many varieties of sulfates, but sodium lauryl sulfate (SLS), sodium ammonium sulfate (ALS), and sodium laureth sulfate (SLES) are the ones most commonly used in personal care products. Sulfates can be found in everything from facial cleansers and toothpaste to the heavy de-greasing agents used to clean the floor in a mechanic's garage. Even in diluted amounts, these sulfates can be irritating to your scalp, skin, and hair. Have you ever gotten shampoo in your eyes? If your eyes burned, sulfates were most likely the culprit.

Your hair needs oil for protection and sulfates strip away that oil, leading to dryness, split ends, fly-aways and dullness. Shampoos with sulfates remove the hair's natural and protective oil and cause unnecessary damage. Sulfates in shampoo also fade hair color. To help maintain the vibrancy and intensity of colored hair, opt for sulfate-free shampoos. There is also frightening evidence that suggests sulfates may harm the immune system and cause serious skin damage. A study performed by Exogenous Dermatology suggests that SLS is a "corrosive irritant" to the skin. It appears that sulfates exert their damage by stripping your skin of protective oils and moisture.[5]

Sneaky Surfactants

Skin cleansers containing sulfates (and/or other harsh surfactants) can lead to dry skin and make it more prone to redness, itching, and irritation. Surfactants are harsh on the skin and hair, and strip the skin of what's known as the acid mantle. The acid mantle refers to the thin barrier of natural oils and desirable dead skin cells that protects the skin from the elements. Surfactants strip the acid mantle away, leaving the skin exposed and vulnerable. Moreover, this stripping effect kicks your skin's oil production into high gear as a protective mechanism, meaning that harsh cleansers actually increase oil production. When the hair, scalp or skin is stripped of natural protective oils, numerous problems arise. Keep in mind that dry skin often leads to premature aging.

Surfactants, including sulfates, are added to produce the lather that we assume means our cleanser is working. However, all of those bubbles spell trouble for our skin and hair. The more high-foaming bubbles or surfactants in a shampoo or cleanser, the more damage may occur. Less lifting and stripping agents means a happier and healthier scalp, skin, and hair. Too many bubbles just get us in trouble!

The Three Pesky Ps

Parabens

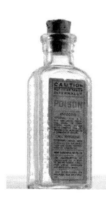

Parabens are a class of chemicals commonly used as preservatives in personal care products such as shampoos, moisturizers, toothpastes, and cosmetics to extend shelf life and prevent the growth of mold and bacteria. The cosmetics industry insists that parabens (which are approved for use by the FDA) are safe. However, many experts firmly disagree.

The current popularity of parabens is most likely based on the fact that they are much cheaper than some newer types of preservatives. This sadly takes precedence over safety in too many cases. Recent studies have brought the issue to the forefront when reports surfaced claiming measurable concentrations of six different parabens have been identified in biopsy samples from breast tumors. The link between parabens and breast cancer is one worthy of concern since these chemicals have been shown to mimic estrogen, a hormone known to play a leading role in breast cancer. So, if a woman has or is prone to an estrogen-dependent illness such as breast cancer or endometriosis, these chemicals are best avoided.

In a study conducted at the University of Reading, British molecular biologist Philippa Darbre found that the ester-bearing form of the parabens found in tumors indicated that their source was a substance applied to the skin, such as underarm deodorant, cream, or body spray. Darbre stated further that the results helped to explain why up to 60 percent of all breast tumors are found in just one-fifth of the breast – the upper-outer quadrant, nearest the underarm.[4]

While this single study shows that there may be a link between parabens and breast tumors, some argue further studies are needed to prove that parabens actually cause breast cancer. However, it supports the likelihood that there is a link between the two. Isn't that enough? As breast cancer accounts for a large percentage of cancers in women, further investigations into the levels of parabens and where they are found in the body should be conducted. While current studies do not definitively link their use with cancerous tumors, neither do studies demonstrate that parabens are safe. The long-term health effects of exposure to parabens have yet to be conclusively proven, so it's a good idea to avoid them. Avoid any ingredient that contains the word paraben ie: propylparaben, butylparaben, methylparaben, isopropyl-paraben, and others.

Phthalates

Phthalates are used to enhance or prolong the fragrance of a cosmetic product. They are commonly found in perfumes, lotions, hair treatment products and nail polish. Phthalates can irritate the nasal passages, cause skin irritation, and even cause contact dermatitis. If you've ever suffered a headache from a perfume or from strong smelling hair or beauty products, phthalates may have been the sneaky culprit. The worst part is that manufacturers are not always required to list phthalates on their product labels, even though these chemicals have been linked to cancer and birth defects. Since there is no way of knowing for sure if a product contains phthalates, it is wise to select only natural, unmodified products that use essential oils and plant extracts as fragrance rather than synthetic chemicals.

Petrochemicals

These sneaky substances are derived from petroleum, so some argue they are natural. The truth is they are anything but natural. They are created using a chemical process that negatively impacts the environment and alters the molecular structure of the chemicals (similar to that which occurs in the production of processed foods). Petrochemicals or petrochemical byproducts are commonly found in products like shampoos, conditioners, mascara, moisturizers, and lip balms. The most well-known members of the petrochemical family include mineral oil, petrolatum, and petroleum jelly. Less familiar names include propylene and butylene glycol, along with polyethylene glycol esters (PEGs), but the list goes on and on. These petroleum-derived personal care ingredients have the potential to cause skin irritation, clogged pores, and allergic reactions such as skin redness and hives in addition to other harmful effects.

Scary derivatives of propylene glycol called polyethylene glycol esters, or PEGs, are made via an ethoxylation process of propylene glycol. This process releases dangerous levels of a toxic compound known as dioxin. Dioxin is a known hormone disruptor and carcinogen. PEGs are widely used in beauty care products as thickeners, softeners, solvents, and penetration enhancers. It is highly advisable to avoid all of these pesky p's.

Remember, the skin is the largest of all organs and needs to function optimally. So, toss those petrochemicals. They don't belong on (or in) your body! There are many products available that don't contain such questionable ingredients.

Dimethicone and Other Sneaky Silicones

Dimethicone is a type of silicone oil that is widely used in skincare products such as moisturizers to treat or prevent dry, rough skin. Dimethicone is one of several silicone oils that is used to add a silky texture to a product, as well as to form a protective barrier on the skin to help retain moisture. The silky smooth feeling these chemicals offer makes consumers love these products, but only because they don't know the real deal. This type of ingredient is often referred to as "occlusive" because it seals in moisture and protects the skin or hair from the elements, as well as from trans-epidermal water loss (TEWD). However, many vegetable oils and botanical ingredients can offer the same properties without the negative side effects of silicone oils.

What is Silicone?

Silicone is any of the polymeric organic silicon compounds obtained as oils, greases, or plastics and used especially for water-resistant and heat-resistant lubricants, varnishes, binders, and electric insulators. Ew!

Manufacturers claim that dimethicone is safe to use because its molecules are too large to enter the pores of the skin. However, studies have found that dimethicone can have negative effects on the body. Dimethicone forms a layer on the skin that wraps anything and everything beneath it including impurities, bacteria, and water that can lead to pimples, bumps and blackheads. In some cases, some products containing dimethicone may cause more skin dryness and irritation as well as itching and redness. Silicone oils like dimethicone are common causes of contact dermatitis and other forms of skin irritation.

Dimethicone and other silicone ingredients are also used in hair care products to add shine and reduce frizz. Silicones coat the surface of hair and lubricate it, making the hair shinier and improving combing and detangling to lessen hair loss and breakage. However, its occlusive property can cause pimples, scalp irritation, and in sensitive individuals, difficulty breathing and swelling of the face or mouth.

Here is a list of some of the many forms of silicone derivatives to watch for on ingredient lists:

- Cyclomethicone
- PEG-12 dimethicone
- Phenyl trimethicone
- Amodimethicone
- Dimethicone copolyol
- Trimethylsiloxyamodimethicone
- Dimethiconol
- PEG-7 dimethicone
- Polysilicone-9
- Divinyl-dimethicone
- Dimethicone copolymer
- Silicone quaternium-8
- PEG-PPG-18/18 dimethicone
- Methicone
- Divinyldimethicone
- Cyclopentasiloxane
- Cyclohexasiloxane

With modern advances in skincare formulations, these sneaky silicones are *not* needed for healthy skin and hair.

Fragrances, Formaldehyde and Other Funky Crap

A rainbow of colors and aromatic fragrances lure you to the cosmetic counters at retail stores. And with good reason, they smell wonderful! But how? While the displays look pretty, many are hiding some very ugly facts. Underneath the fancy packaging many beauty products are filled with synthetic dyes, artificial ingredients, and toxic fragrances.

According to a 1986 report by the Committee on Science & Technology in the U.S. House of Representatives, 95 percent of chemicals in perfumes and fragranced products are synthetic chemicals derived from petroleum. Some of these chemicals are known to have negative health consequences, mainly due to effects on the central nervous system.[6]

Synthetic fragrances are often difficult to pinpoint. There are hundreds of ingredients that are considered synthetic fragrances. A good indication that a product has one or more of these smelly culprits is when the label simply reads "fragrance." Synthetic fragrances can cause nausea, skin irritation, headache, dizziness, coughing, and vomiting.

While synthetic fragrances often smell heavy and unnatural, essential oils and plant-derived hydrosols have a pleasantly rich scent with added aromatherapy benefits. Cosmetics, bath products, and skincare products can be purchased with hydrosols or pure essential oils. Your nose may not always know the difference, though, so it's important to do your homework.

Examples of popular essential oils used in a variety of skin care, hair care and beauty products include: lavender, lemon, tea tree, grapefruit, patchouli, frankincense, rose, and orange. However, even some product manufacturers use synthetic counterparts of natural essential oils because they are a fraction of the cost. So, just because the label says "lavender" doesn't mean it's pure lavender. Use caution here and seek a reputable manufacturer.

Formaldehyde and Urea Compounds – These ingredients may be found in all kinds of products, including fertilizer, pressed wood and diuretics, plus skin, nail and hair care products. DMDM hydantoin, diazolidinyl urea and imidazolidinyl urea are commonly used preservatives that can release formaldehyde. These ingredients have long been used in cosmetics as preservatives, or in conjunction with a preservative to inhibit mold and bacteria formation. Exposure to formaldehyde and/or formaldehyde releasers may cause joint pain, headaches, skin and scalp irritation, chronic fatigue, and more. Ureas may also cause dermatitis in some individuals. They are also considered possible carcinogens. With so many other options, you should avoid these ingredients and select less risky alternatives. Also, beware of Brazilian hair blowouts that use formaldehyde.

Synthetic colors are used to make cosmetics more eye-catching, but when you see the color labeled with a letter and number such as FD&C Red No. 6, you should stay away. Synthetic dyes are used in makeup, lipstick, hair dyes, and even body products such as moisturizers. While the colors might appear vibrant, they could be carcinogenic.

Alternatively, there are natural ingredients that can be used to add color to natural skincare products and makeup, including essential oils, fruit and vegetable juices, carrot oil, and even beet extract. Non-chemical colorants are used often in mineral makeup brands.

Steer clear of synthetic fragrance, formaldehyde, and other funky-sounding fillers to be safe rather than sorry.

Hydroquinone Belongs Down the Throne!

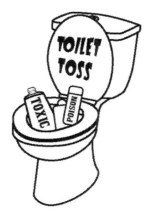

Ever wish for a brighter, lighter or more even skin tone? Looking to reduce age spots, scarring and discoloration? Be careful what you ask for! Many skin-lightening creams and serums contain hydroquinone, a cosmetic bleaching agent that suppresses the production of melanin (the pigment that creates a tan), thus reducing the skin's natural protection against damaging ultraviolet (UV) radiation. Hydroquinone penetrates the skin and may cause irreversible damage to connective tissue including skin, which may also contribute to premature aging.

According to the U.S. Environmental Protection Agency, laboratory studies have found an increased skin tumor incidence in mice treated dermally with hydroquinone.[7] Even though the FDA has yet to label this chemical as a known carcinogen for humans, a potential risk has been identified. Hydroquinone has also been found to cause skin photosensitivity (greater sensitivity to the sun's effects) resulting in rashes, blotches, and discoloration when exposed to the sun. Because this chemical can be absorbed through the skin and into the bloodstream, there may also a risk of liver and kidney damage. In simplest terms, these chemicals are toxic and possibly in ways we are not even aware of yet. An ingredient that carries such serious risks shouldn't be used on your skin, especially when alternatives exist that achieve the same result yet are safe, natural and without risks!

Some non-toxic skin lightening and brightening ingredients include: licorice root, lemon, turmeric, vitamin C, and vitamin B3 (niacinimide). Look for these natural ingredients when choosing a skincare product, and limit your sun exposure and inflammation to avoid future challenges.

Why take the chance with all the risks? To the throne with hydroquinone!

Beware of Benzoyl Peroxide

Commonly used in the treatment of acne, benzoyl peroxide, or BPO, dries up oil and kills anaerobic bacteria by flooding them with oxygen. Flushing the pores with this popular material may be effective, but according to the Material Safety Data Sheet (MSDS), benzoyl peroxide is a possible tumor promoter. *Say what??* In high concentrations, it may act as a mutagen and produce DNA damage in human cells. It is toxic if inhaled, harmful if swallowed, and benzoyl peroxide is also a skin, eye, and respiratory irritant.[8]

BPO can also dry out skin, stain towels, sheets, and clothing, and even bleach hair and eyebrows. It is not recommended for sensitive skin or for use around the eyes, lips or mouth. Don't believe it? Manufacturers are now required to list this on the labels. It can also easily remove the top layer of your skin, increasing sun sensitivity and potential UV damage. In addition, a small percentage of the population is allergic to benzoyl peroxide. I happen to be one of them, and trust me it was painful!

Last Call for Alcohol?

There are various types of alcohols used in the personal care industry for a variety of functions. While some are beneficial, others are not. Overuse of *certain* types of alcohols is very drying and can strip the skin of its natural protective lipids (or fats). In addition, some alcohols have chemicals added to them that may be harmful. It's important that you are able to distinguish the beneficial alcohol-based skincare ingredients from the ones that damage your skin.

Alcohol, otherwise known as "ethanol," is a naturally derived ingredient commonly sourced from corn, wheat and sugar cane. This is your common drinkable alcohol, while denatured or specially denatured (SD) alcohol is also ethanol but has a chemical added to it rendering it undrinkable. Methanol and Isopropyl alcohols are often sold as "rubbing alcohol" and are commonly referred to as denatured or specially denatured. These alcohols are the ones to avoid. Alcohol *may* also be "naturally denatured" which is not harmful to the skin when incorporated into a finished product properly, but this is not the most common method.

Then we have the alcohols known as "fatty alcohols." They may be extracted from natural sources such as coconuts, palm, etc. In the cosmetics industry, they are used as emulsifiers, emollients and as thickeners in the formulation of creams, among other things. These alcohols are generally considered safe for the skin, although they should still be used with caution and in moderation.

A History of Alcohol in Cosmetics

So how did we end up with so many alcohols in beauty products anyway? Specially denatured alcohols were first used in skincare products because they were a cheap solvent. They were used in toners (astringents) and in cold creams to break the surface tension of the petrolatum so the cream wouldn't leave a greasy after-feel. Two things made people think the products were effectively cleaning the skin: 1) they could feel it working, and 2) they could see what they thought was dirt or grime on the cotton used to apply the product. In reality, what they were really looking at was the natural lipids that had been stripped from the skin's protective barrier layer.

Over the years, knowledge in the science of skin care has evolved, and we now know that it is important to keep this protective barrier layer intact. To do this, you should avoid skincare products that contain any of the following aggravating alcohols: SD (specially denatured) alcohols including rubbing alcohol, isopropyl alcohol, and methyl alcohol (methanol).

These alcohols are drying and can strip the skin of its natural barrier layer (known as the acid mantle), dehydrating the underlying skin cells and reducing its protective mechanism. This is why alcohol-based facial toners designed to reduce oiliness of the skin seem to work (for the first few weeks) but later lead to bigger problems. The oils eventually return because the purpose of these oils on the skin is to protect vital organs from bacteria and chemical invasion. Alcohols are only beneficial to the skin when they are free of harmful chemical additives and when combined with the right amount of carrier oils, humectants, and/or butters.

SD alcohols can also cause blood vessel dilation, inflammation, premature aging, fine lines and wrinkles, and may interfere with your body's ability to absorb certain vitamins. They cannot be ingested and should not be absorbed by the skin because they can create a vicious cycle of damage, and other skin problems.

However, some alcohols are considered safe for use. Coconut, cetearyl, stearyl, and cetyl alcohols (plant derived) are a few of them. Commonly used as emulsifiers, they bind water and oil and are found in conditioners, creams, and lotions. In addition, grain, grape, and sugar cane alcohols are commonly used to extract the active constituents from raw plant materials and are used in the creation of botanical extracts or herbal tinctures. These alcohols are often used in organic beauty products. Benzyl alcohol is yet another naturally occurring alcohol derived from plant sources, and therefore present in some essential oils, but it may also be synthesized. This version is what you want to be wary of.

The No Bull Beauty Solution is to only use safe alcohols, in moderation, and trust your skin when it tells you it's dry or irritated - then back off! Remember: you shouldn't have to feel your skincare product to know it's working!

Tricky Triclosan

Antibacterial, anti-viral, and anti-fungal agents are good, aren't they? Though they might sound beneficial, these products could be hiding something I refer to as tricky triclosan.

So what is it? Triclosan is used in pesticides, insulation, textiles, plastics and mattresses to slow the growth of mildew, fungi, and bacteria. It is also utilized in (you guessed it) personal care products such as soaps, toothpastes, shaving cream, mouthwashes, hand sanitizers, dish detergents, and deodorants. At one time the FDA claimed triclosan was not hazardous to humans. More recently, they have decided that triclosan should be reviewed further to determine if it poses health risks. For starters, researchers at Tufts University School of Medicine report that, Triclosan is capable of forcing the emergence of "super bugs" that it cannot kill.[9] Eww! This would explain why Triclosan was first registered by the EPA in 1969…as a pesticide!

Other studies have indicated that triclosan may also affect the endocrine system and fetal development. In addition, triclosan may be no more effective at getting rid of germs than soap and water. So, why would anyone use this in his or her products?! Always check the label and avoid products containing triclosan.

The Skinny on Sunscreen

SPF, or Sun Protection Factor, is the measurement of sunscreen's ability to prevent harmful UV rays from damaging the skin. SPFs are classified as OTC (over-the-counter) drugs by the FDA. These products must undergo efficacy testing to ensure they offer the level of protection they claim to.

According to the American Cancer Society, skin cancer is the most common type of cancer, with more than 3.5 million cases diagnosed each year.[10] As discussed earlier, skin is the largest organ in the human body. It's also one of the most important so we absolutely must protect it!

Inquiring Minds Want to Know!

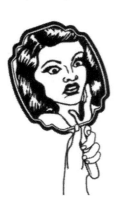 Are the ingredients in SPFs more of a threat than overexposure to sun when it comes to deadly skin cancer and skin damage? Many people pick up sunscreen products without even considering the safety of the ingredients. Since this is something you plan to rub into your skin from head to toe to protect it, it seems reasonable to make sure the ingredients are *actually* safe.

Even if you don't lie on the beach, it's a good idea to arm yourself daily with sun protection when you are driving, hiking, biking, or playing sports. Even if it seems cloudy, the sun's harmful UV rays can still penetrate the windshield of your car and windows and make their way straight to your skin. Don't think you are not at risk during the winter months either, as these rays are present all year round no matter where you live.

The sun has two types of ultraviolet rays that directly affect your skin: UVA (ultraviolet A) and UVB (ultraviolet B). UVA rays tan the skin and also penetrate glass windows and light clothing, while reaching the deeper layers of your skin. UVB rays are absorbed through the uppermost layers of your skin, cause tanning or sunburn and have been linked to two types of skin cancer, squamous-cell and basal-cell carcinomas. Although many people believe having a tan looks healthy, the tan is actually an indication that your skin has experienced a cellular injury. Skin challenges such as wrinkles, blemishes, blotches, and rough texture are caused by UVA cellular damage. So remember, UVA and UVB rays accelerate aging. More importantly, overexposure to UVA rays can jeopardize your skin and make it prone to melanoma – the deadliest type of skin cancer.

The solution? To prevent accelerated aging, skin injury, and skin cancer, make sure to use a sunscreen that offers both UVA and UVB protection. Opt for a product that is labeled "broad spectrum" as these products will protect from both types of UV rays (UVA/UVB). Any other type is simply not protecting your skin fully. Many sunscreens claim an SPF 50 or higher, but new FDA regulations require sunscreens to have a maximum of 50 since a higher SPF does not always mean much more protection. Bottom line: A broad spectrum sunscreen with an SPF of 30 will provide higher levels of protection than a "full-spectrum" sunscreen with an SPF of 50. Since all of this is very confusing, the FDA is mandating many changes to SPF labeling in years to come. Thank goodness!

What the Hey! Sunscreen and Sunblock are Not the Same?

What's the difference between a sunblock and a sunscreen? Even though these terms are used interchangeably, they are very different when it comes to ingredients. Sunblock *blocks* your skin from the sun, while sunscreen *absorbs UV rays*. Sunscreens that contain toxic chemical SPF ingredients often irritate the eyes and also cause major skin irritation.

Sunblocks on the other hand often have a slightly thicker consistency and remain on the skin for a longer period of time. Instead of chemical SPFs, sunblock uses "physical blocks" such as titanium dioxide or zinc oxide, which are more natural and less sensitizing. When these types of blocks are applied, UV rays are deflected before your skin absorbs them. While there is no perfect solution, non-nanoparticle zinc oxide is my SPF ingredient of choice. Nanoparticle mineral SPFs were developed to minimize the white pastey appearance that occurred with traditional mineral sunblocks. However, these pesky nano (tiny) particles can enter the bloodstream and may be hazardous to your health. Mineral sunblocks offer a better option than chemical screens; just make sure to avoid annoying nanoparticles.

Royal Oils

Many oils also offer natural sun protection, including the oil your skin produces, (yet another reason not to strip your skin via harsh cleansers and ingredients). However, you would not know what level of protection you are getting so don't rely on that alone. Natural oils derived from berries, along with potent antioxidants and omega-rich ingredients are making their way into the future of sunscreen technology. We may already be there by the time you read this. Otherwise, for now a combination of a physical sunblock with non-nanoparticle zinc oxide and sun protective clothing like a long-sleeve breathable shirt and hat offer the best solution while newer options are being tested. The terms "sunscreen" and "sunblock" are used interchangeably today, so be sure to read the labels for your preferred ingredients before buying.

And always remember: for the most protection apply your SPF thirty minutes before going outdoors, and immediately after exposure to excessive sweating or water. It is best to reapply sunblock every 2 hours. Select a broad spectrum sunblock with at least a 30 SPF. Since they are typically chemical-free, the mineral based sunblocks are also a better choice for those with sensitive or reactive skin. You should, however, read the label to see what other sneaky ingredients may be present.

Scary Chemical Sunscreens

According to studies performed by the Centers for Disease Control, 97 percent of Americans use sunscreens that contain an ingredient known as oxybenzone.[11] This ingredient has been linked to allergies, hormone disruption, and cellular damage. One study revealed that oxybenzone is linked to low birth weight in baby girls whose mothers were exposed to it during pregnancy. As harmful ingredients are often absorbed via the bloodstream, do your best to protect yourself.

Be aware of some sneaky suspect sunscreen ingredients such as:

- Oxybenzone
- Octinoxate
- Octocrylene
- Para amino benzoic acid
- Octyl salicylate
- PABA and PAGA esters
- Cinnamates
- Avobenzone
- Homosalate
- Trolamine salicylate
- Octocrylene
- Dioxybenzone
- Phenylbenziimidazole
- Cinoxate
- Retinyl palmitate
- Homosalate
- Menthyl anthranilate
- Sulisobenzone
- Nano-particles
- Padimate and, of course, all toxic preservatives

Whew! If that is as overwhelming for you as for me, simply copy, print, and take this list with you when shopping.[12]

Natural Ways to Protect Your Skin From Sun Damage

A diet rich in high-antioxidant whole citrus fruits, tomatoes, berries, raw cocoa, green and red tea, along with dark leafy green vegetables is another way to protect your skin from sun damage.

Vitamins A and C are essential, as skin cells utilize these antioxidant vitamins to regulate light absorption and protect against overexposure. Proper nutrition is always a great way to protect your body from the inside out!

In summary, to keep from stripping your skin of protective oils, you should avoid harsh products and always use a non-toxic broad spectrum SPF, eat an antioxidant-rich diet, and try to evade direct exposure to the sun during the hours of 10 a.m. and 4 p.m. Play it safe. Protect your skin 365 days a year!

Are Sunless Tans Really Worth It?

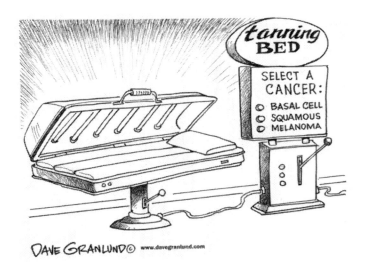

Most dermatologists warn against indoor tanning and the National Institutes of Health has declared radiation a carcinogen. According to the World Health Association, no one under 18 should use a tanning bed, under any circumstances. The Center for Disease

Control (CDC) and FDA encourage folks to avoid using sunlamps and tanning beds (or booths) because of these potential hazards. Some sources state that UV tanners are more likely to get melanoma than people who never go to tanning beds. Is it not time these things are banned?

Some self-tanners may also be hazardous. The active chemical used to provide a tanned appearance in popular "spray-on" tans, dihydroxyacetone (DHA) has the potential to cause DNA damage, according to some medical experts. [13] A concern is that DHA may enter the lungs, aiding systemic absorption. Adverse effects that have been reported include coughing, rashes, and dizziness. A mask and good ventilation is recommended but not always available. Opting for hand-applied self-tanning products like creams, lotions, mousses and gels might be a better choice if you *have to* use a self-tanner at all. Another issue with some self-tanners is the presence of synthetic fragrances and phthalates (amongst other things), so read the labels. In addition, these colorants can appear blotchy or uneven and also leave streaks if not applied correctly or if you have dry, flaky skin. It's not exactly the ideal way to get the glowing tan that most people are looking for. And is it worth it?

One potential alternative is to eat a diet rich in carotenoids, which are clinically proven to naturally enhance your skin tone. Moreover, carotenoids have a myriad of other benefits, including potent antioxidant and anti-inflammatory effects. Sounds like a better deal to me!

Poisonous Polish? PU!

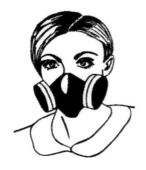

When it comes to beauty, a sun-kissed tan, luscious locks, and beautiful nails are all desirable. However, these things are not always free of harmful effects, as previously discussed. One of the biggest headaches when you polish your nails is that dreadful smell. PU! If regular nail polish smells that noxious, can you imagine what it might be doing to your body systems or to the environment? If you've ever asked yourself "Should I really be putting this stinky stuff on my nails, and in the air I'm breathing?" the answer is no, and there are alternatives! Some of the newer, less toxic nail polish brands avoid the use of three major questionable ingredients including formaldehyde, toluene, and dibutyl phthalate (DBP). These icky chemicals are linked to a host of problems ranging from skin irritation to illnesses when used in large doses or over time. These toxins are what make nail polish stink.

Choosing non-toxic nail polish also means you don't have to use the nasty nail polish remover with additional toxins such as acetone and phthalates, which can disrupt your endocrine system. Another HUGE problem is flushing toxins in nail polish and nail polish removers. They contaminate the water supply, causing all kinds of problems including the destruction of ecosystems and marine life. So what does a girl have to do to get pretty nails *and* be health and eco-conscious?

There are newer, safer nail polish options that are free of carcinogens and are often water-based. Most of them are odorless, so you don't get a headache, breathe toxic fumes, or offend the people you live with. Most non-toxic nail polish is easily removed with non-toxic removers, and some types even peel off. The lasting power is excellent and comparable to those wonderful yet noxious nail polishes. Non-toxic nail polish is also available in a rainbow of cool colors. It's definitely good stuff and the girly way to go green!

If you love salon pampering, you can also bring your green essentials with you. Why not? Just hand it to them and say, "No caca on my cuticles, please!"

Pore-Clogging Crap

Did you know that many face creams, serums and even cleansers contain pore-clogging crap? Here you are trying to cleanse and moisturize your face, and instead you're just clogging your pores so your skin can't absorb the good ingredients? It's time to scrap the stuff that clogs your pores, so the good stuff can get in there and reveal the radiant healthy skin you desire!

So What Are Some of the 'Bad Boys' You Should Avoid?

These ingredients include, but are not limited to:

- Silicones
- Mineral oil
- Isopropyl myristate

- Myristyl myristate
- Octyl myristate
- Isopropyl alcohol
- Hexadecyl alcohol
- Octyl palmitate
- Sodium chloride

Dizzy yet? If you are not a chemist, this is sure to make your head spin. Print the list and take it shopping with you. One of the worst offenders is isopropyl myristate (ice-a-propyl-meer-estate) so be on the lookout for that bad boy, as it sneaks its way into a lot of products. And don't be fooled by Mother Nature, as even some popular ingredients like wheat germ oil and cocoa butter can be too much for acne-prone skin.

Body lotions, creams, cleansers, shampoo, hairspray, deodorant, body butters, and makeup can all contain pore-clogging crap, so check those labels!

Other Pore-Clogging Crap

Hair Products - If you suffer from breakouts or irritation around the hairline or scalp, your shampoo, conditioner or styling products may contain some pore-clogging or comedogenic (another word for pore-clogging) culprits. Did you ever consider that if hairspray can create a hard film on the hair, it may do the same to your skin? Voila - clogged pores!

Makeup - There is a whole plethora of ingredients that cause clogged pores and blemishes so consider selecting high-quality mineral makeup and try to use less if you are prone to breakouts.

Toothpaste - If you break out around your mouth, or have any redness or inflammation, your toothpaste may be the culprit! Perioral dermatitis is something I see often in my practice. The mere suggestion to "ditch the toothpaste" and try a sulfate and chemical-free solution often solves the problem. Simply washing your face after tooth brushing versus prior is another way to be sure to remove any trace of icky ingredient residue.

If you thought only an acne sufferer need worry, think again. Avoidance of pore clogging ingredients is easier than fixing the problems that can result from using them.

Does Your Deodorant Stink?

Knowing the difference between a deodorant and an antiperspirant is important. Don't you want to know if the ingredients in the products you put under your arms are doing harm or good?

Deodorant simply eliminates unpleasant body odors, as it is just a "de-odor-izer." However some deodorants contain synthetic fragrance, dyes and even irritating chemicals, making them sensitizing or allergy-producing.

Antiperspirant on the other hand, actually interferes with the body's natural cooling process and prevents perspiration. Antiperspirants often contain aluminum-based compounds as the active ingredient. Antiperspirants temporarily *plug the sweat duct* and stop the flow of perspiration to the surface of your skin. Some research suggests that applying antiperspirant near the breast can cause estrogen-like hormonal effects. Estrogen, as we know, may promote the growth of breast cancer cells (a serious risk for us ladies).

So is Aluminum a Toxin? The Agency for Toxic Substances and Disease Registry reports that "exposure to high levels of aluminum may result in respiratory and neurological problems."[14] Now what exactly is *high*? Does that mean repeated use over many years, or even weeks?

Some studies even suggest a link between aluminum toxicity and Alzheimer's disease.[15][16] While there is not enough evidence to prove this link, I recommend you avoid it. Aluminum (as well as most antiperspirant ingredients) will actually penetrate the skin and enter your bloodstream where it is said to have the most risks for long-term health issues.

Toss Terrible Talc!

You will also want to be sure to avoid the ingredient talc in your deodorant, body powder and cosmetic products. Studies on talc have revealed it to be similar in structure to asbestos, a well known cancer causing agent. *What the…?* Talc has also been associated with lung cancer and pneumonia, as the tiny particles in this terrible toxin can easily enter the lungs and cause inflammation. This ingredient is scary!

Talc particles can move through the reproductive system and even become imbedded in the ovarian lining. If that is not enough for you, researchers discovered that women with ovarian cancer were more frequent users of talcum powder in the genital area than were healthy women.[17]

Your pets and children are not immune to this toxin either. Exposing any living thing to this carcinogen is unnecessary and dangerous. Toss the talc and talcum powder today!

Other trends: Botulinum toxin (also known as Botox®, Dysport®, and other names) is another popular treatment for controlling excessive perspiration. This requires visits to a physician a few times per year to have the sweat glands injected with this product or other similar products. Side effects of Botox injections may include headache, nausea, and pain. It takes a lot of product and needles and is costly, not to mention temporary. In extreme cases, men and women are actually having sweat glands removed – ouch!

So what do you do to control stinky body odor safely and affordably? There are many natural non-toxic options including crystal deodorants, therapeutic essential oil blends, and even eating body odor-blocking herbs, such as parsley, oregano, thyme, mint and detoxifying foods like limes! Avoiding processed foods can also help. The high amount of salt, sugar and hydrogenated oils can irritate the stomach and trigger the production of body odor. A magnesium deficiency may also contribute to ferocious funk levels, so adding foods rich in this nutrient such as almonds and oatmeal can help. Spinach and other leafy greens contain minerals including magnesium, and also deliver odor-fighting chlorophyll!

Heavy Metal Makeup Doesn't Rock!

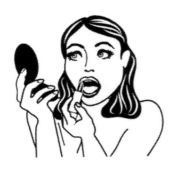

Many of us do not give a second thought to what we are applying in the way of makeup. All we know is that it improves our self-esteem and appearance, but there is much more to it than that. There are certain facts every woman should know before applying cosmetics.

Toxic metals that are commonly found in makeup include, but are not limited to lead, cobalt, nickel, and chromium.

The FDA allows the use of **mercury** compounds in eye makeup at concentrations levels up to 65 parts per million. The preservative **thimerosol** found in some mascaras (as well as some vaccinations) also contains mercury.

Serious Health Risks

Mercury is one of the most toxic substances on Earth and is associated with a host of health concerns including allergic reactions, skin irritation, toxicity, neurological damage, bioaccumulation and environmental harm. Mercury readily passes into the body through the skin, so regular use of products containing mercury results in exposure. The FDA has issued a public warning against mercury in products, although there are still many products containing mercury on the market today.[18]

Look Out for Lead in Your Lipstick

Did you know that the average woman consumes 7 pounds of lipstick in her lifetime?[19] Repeated licking of the lips and eating while wearing these crazy colorful cosmetics eventually means you are ingesting some every time you wear it. And that adds up. What you may not know is that it's not just a little lipstick you're ingesting; it may be toxic heavy metals. *Woah!*

Heavy metal lipstick is a major problem. The Database for Safe Cosmetics recently revealed that lipsticks contain an alarming level of lead. Recently the FDA tested 400 lipsticks for lead content. On average, lead content in lipsticks was 1.07 ppm, with some containing up to 3.07 ppm. The FDA indicated that these lipsticks were in the acceptable range.[20] The point is that any amount of lead in lipstick should not be acceptable.

Why? Over time, lead exposure is toxic and poisonous to the body. It builds up in soft tissue such as the brain, liver, kidneys, and bone marrow, along with your teeth and bones. In children, permanent damage has been reported along with serious learning disabilities, stunted growth, and other negative side effects.[21] In severe cases with high blood concentrations, children have been become severely ill.

Lead permeates our everyday life in corners we might not expect. Let's consider a few unexpected things that might be exposing you to lead.

In addition to some lipsticks, lead acetate is found in "progressive" hair colors that are applied over a period of time to gradually change hair color. That means extended exposure to lead. "Natural" hair coloring options like henna may sound better, but henna products usually contain metallic elements as well. Don't trade in your silvery highlights for "real" metallic ones.

You may also be ingesting lead when you eat. Many fish contain mercury and lead, so it is important to know where the fish you consume are harvested. If they contain high toxic levels, you should avoid them. Lead actually exists in nature in abundance, but it is anything but safe in and on our bodies.

Another source of lead at the dinner table is lead stemware. With continued use, toxic levels of lead can build up in your system. Steer clear of lead stemware and use plain glassware instead. The cost of brilliance is way too high! Be safe, and avoid the lead in your life.

Mineral Makeup Madness

Mineral makeup is presently one of the hottest cosmetic trends. We often think of minerals as a good thing, but while mineral makeup may not contain parabens and petrochemicals, some (not all) can contain nanoparticles. These minute particles can be irritating for some wearers, causing inflammation and other problems as a result of ongoing inhalation. Keep an eye out for *bismuth oxychloride*, a common makeup ingredient. While it does not irritate most women, it can cause acne or irritation in some individuals.

Pros and Cons of Mineral Makeup

Pros:

1. **Mineral makeup often naturally contains UV protectants** and helps defend skin against harmful, cancer-causing rays. It's also often water-resistant and stays decent after a brief swim.

2. **Mineral makeup has a light appearance,** which is convenient as you can build layers to get the exact coverage and texture you want. Only you know it is makeup!

3. **These cosmetics are safer, and non-comedogenic,** even though some of the ingredients (as with anything) may irritate certain skin types. This means they are also less likely to break you out or clog pores like the alternatives.

Cons:

1. **It is not ideal for asthma and allergy sufferers.** The loose powder may aggravate these conditions and pose potential health concerns. Some experts suggest long-term use of mica particles found in mineral makeup can cause inflammation or irritation and lead to lung problems.

2. **Natural doesn't necessarily mean non-irritating.** Some mineral makeups contain nanoparticles and sensitizing ingredients such as bismuth oxychloride. They can irritate the skin. Try to avoid them.

3. **The powder can settle into deep wrinkles.** If the skin lacks hydration and is not exfoliated, powder can actually settle into these areas and make wrinkles appear more

pronounced. Who wants to enhance wrinkles? Using a good moisturizer prior to application can help prevent this.

4. **Big con.** The loose powder options are a bit messy and may fill the atmosphere contributing to both health and environmental issues.

In general, mineral makeup often contains less toxins then traditional cosmetics, which makes it a better option. If you select to use mineral makeup, consider the pressed powder option to both minimize the mess and the potential for particle dispersion in the environment. Whether you opt for loose or pressed powders, to play it safe, apply it in a well-ventilated area or by an open window. Of course, you also want to avoid the irritating additives along with anything else that sounds suspicious.

Funky-Fresh Preservatives

Preservatives are necessary ingredients to keep cosmetics and skincare products safe and free from mold, bacteria and other harmful microorganisms. But as we discussed previously, the safety of some of these funky-fresh chemicals is questionable. We reviewed parabens and formaldehyde donors earlier, and unfortunately, the list of crappy chemical preservatives simply goes on and on. While some preservatives are highly controversial, natural and organic preservative systems do exist, although they may cost more in some cases. However, on occasion, manufacturers slip some other bad boys into "natural" products thinking the name sounds benign. Some preservatives have been banned in other countries that are still considered safe in the USA.

So why are preservatives necessary? Just as with food, if a mixed product contains water (or juice, tea, fruit, and other water based ingredients), a preservative is an absolute necessity... yet a potentially irritating or toxic preservative is certainly not. One concern that many manufacturers present in regards to natural preservation is that the shelf life may be limited. While this is not necessarily true, they certainly have the option to create smaller batches, but as this is not always cost effective it's easier and cheaper to toss in the chemical crap. Easier and cheaper doesn't make it right. Personally, I don't want my beauty products hanging around forever. Food is best fresh, and I would argue the same for beauty products. Even the chemical crap should be tossed out regularly as the efficacy of ingredients will diminish over time.

Some of the cutting-edge preservatives today are plant derived and offer incredible efficacy. Often beauty products require additional ingredients such as antioxidants to prevent rancidity of ingredients, or pH modifiers to prevent irritation to the skin and prevent nasty bugs from growing. Some manufacturers are turning to jars and treatment pumps in an effort to keep dirty hands out of the bottle. Dark tinted bottles are also useful in preventing light from affecting the product's stability, and glass is less likely to absorb the scent and ingredients than plastic. The bottom line is this - preservatives are a necessity just as they are in the food you consume, so let's not take a risk. Would you want bacteria in your eyes? Don't think so! Just seek a reputable manufacturer and avoid the "crap."

2

The Lowdown on Labels

Confusing Label Lingo

Preservatives, emulsifiers, botanical names, fragrances, chemicals, preservatives, SPF numbers, fillers, and funky sounding names make a simple purchase not so simple. What the heck?! Ingredients in cosmetics can be confusing as all get out. It can be difficult to determine what to purchase and what to steer away from. This chapter is here to help.

5 Rules of Thumb for Reading Labels

1. **If it seems too good to be true, it probably is!** Beware of claims that sound too good to be true, and products that claim to be a miracle in a bottle.

2. **Know that "natural" doesn't mean much.** Labeling a product as "natural" or "all-natural" is one of the most abused claims out there so read the entire ingredient list.

3. **Be wary of unnamed fragrances.** The word "fragrance" sounds simple until you realize synthetic fragrances can irritate and/or contain phthalates, (those crappy chemical toxins that negatively impact the neurological and endocrine systems). Real natural essential oils are the better option, but only if you are not sensitive to them.

4. **"Oil free" often misleads.** This claim may appeal to those with oily or blemish-prone skin, but keep in mind that non-oil ingredients often contribute to these problems. And remember that many plant-derived oils can actually treat these problems successfully.

5. **Confusing ingredient names.** Remember, if something sounds benign it may not be and vice versa. Seek a beauty professional's advice to help decipher the ingredients and determine if they are appropriate for your skin type.

Bogus Beauty Claims

Crazy Commercial Claims

When you see commercials claiming "95 percent of women saw an improvement in two to four weeks." Just before saying "WOW," you should consider asking yourself a few of the following questions: How many women did they actually use for the test? What if they only used twenty women? Is that number sufficient to represent the whole population? Did the ages and prior conditions of these women vary, or did they handpick specific ones? And who conducted the study, the company itself or an outside group? This type of efficacy testing is very costly and generally only afforded by major cosmetic manufacturers. That's not to say the product does not offer the results it claims, but results will vary per individual as results depend greatly upon your lifestyle. The best way to know if a product will yield the results you desire is to simply try it yourself! Also beware of before and after photos....if it looks too good to be true, it may just be.

Hypoallergenic and Non-Comedogenic

These terms are used to convey to consumers that if they use a product, they won't experience an allergic reaction or clogged pores (acne). Some of these tests are based on a population sample, meaning that if 50 people are tested without incident, there is no guarantee that number 51 won't have a reaction. The term "oil free" also suggests a non-comedogenic product, however a number of ingredients aside from oils can contribute to skin irritation and breakouts. It is best to always test a product first on a small area, just to know it's safe for you, especially if you are sensitive or prone to breakouts.

Natural is Just a Buzz Word

In trying to make a product appear safe and harmless, some manufacturers loosely use the terms "100% natural," or "all-natural." Don't let these labels comfort you, because they merely mean that there may be one percent of a natural ingredient in the product amongst 99 percent synthetic ingredients. It's true that there are no strict criteria to call a product "natural." Read the labels before you buy. You can always try a product in a small, sensitive area such as behind the ear or inner elbow first to test for irritation or a potential allergic reaction. Just because something is from nature does not guarantee it's safe…consider poison ivy!

Greenwashing Garbage

At one time, "green" products were almost exclusively consumed by true naturalists. Back then huge corporations weren't producing natural or organic versions of their products because the mainstream wasn't interested. Then things changed. Hooray!

People are more informed about the threats that exist in our toxic, chemical-laden lives and as a result more people are looking for natural products that are safe for their family and the environment.

The bad news is that the large corporations that have been successfully selling these toxic products don't necessarily want to change. That would cut into their mega-profits and frankly just be too much work. But on the other hand, they know they are going to lose customers if they don't listen to the consumer's wishes, so these companies often turn to the practice known as "greenwashing."

Greenwashing is the term used to describe a company's attempt to misrepresent a product's real ingredients or processing methods by way of advertising gimmicks. This practice makes a product appear eco-friendly even though in reality, it is still the same conventional, toxic product. This problem has run rampant in the beauty industry in particular because there are no strict regulations on labeling personal care products. It is unfortunate that consumers have to do their own sleuthing to avoid many harmful ingredients!

So, What Can You Do?

The number of greenwashed products on the market is increasing every day. The key is to familiarize yourself with ingredients so you can make informed decisions. With the lack of regulations as we previously reviewed, "all-natural" does not indicate a better product. Just because you purchase it at a natural food store does not mean it is good for you, or good for the planet.

A growing number of products make lofty claims about being eco-friendly, preservative-free, oil-free, natural, cruelty-free, organic, and hypoallergenic, etc. However, many of these claims are unsubstantiated. Bogus beauty claims are cleverly disguised, so do your research and become a conscious consumer that doesn't buy into the Bull!

Stinky INCI Names

The FDA requires that health and beauty product labels use International Nomenclature Cosmetic Ingredient (INCI) names for all ingredients, with the exception of fragrance, which is considered proprietary. INCI names were established to ensure that cosmetic ingredients are consistently listed under the same name from product to product, and in various countries. INCI terminology can make your head spin!

For example, ingredients listed in the scientific Latin names may appear harmful. The scary sounding *Simmondsia chinensis* is actually the very beneficial jojoba seed oil, a naturally derived ingredient offering hydration for skin. *Camellia sinensis* is simply antioxidant-rich green tea. It's all good!

Then there are threatening-sounding formal names that really are bad for you, like sodium laureth sulfate, formaldehyde, and methylparaben, which are all toxic ingredients. These are the stinky ones! The list goes on and on...

Beware of certain ingredients that sound simple. The word "fragrance" seems straightforward until you realize that many fragrances contain nasty chemical compounds from those pesky phthalates. Unless they are made with pure essential oils, many fragrances contain chemical toxins that can have a negative impact on your neurological system.

Here are samples of some ok ingredients, and their INCI names:

- Aloe Barbadensis (Aloe Vera)
- Sodium Bicarbonate (Baking Soda)
- Melissa Officinalis (Lemon Balm)
- Sodium Chloride (Dead Sea Salt)
- Lavandula Angustifolia (Lavender)
- Olea Europaea (Olive Oil)

Don't let your judgment be clouded by confusing INCI names because the English name will likely be present alongside them. If not, you can always contact the manufacturer for more information.

Confused by Cosmeceuticals?

Cosmeceuticals may be a hot buzzword, but what does it mean? It sure sounds promising, but does it mean it's a cosmetic with pharmaceutical-like benefits as you might assume?

Cosmeceuticals are designed to influence the biological function of your skin in order to reduce the appearance of wrinkles, improve skin tone and texture, and deliver nutrients for healthier, younger-looking skin. They are also marketed as "nutraceuticals" or "actives." The FDA does not allow these products to use drug claims so, while a product may in fact offer drug-like benefits, such as acne reduction, healing and hair loss reduction, the label may not indicate it. In this case, the product would be recognized as a "drug" and not a "cosmetic."

Much like standard cosmetics, cosmeceuticals are applied topically to enhance or improve your skin. The common trait among cosmeceuticals is that they contain therapeutic-grade ingredients intended to produce a specific dermatological effect. Ingredients may include vitamins and botanical ingredients such as vitamin C, glycolic acid, green tea, pomegranate extract, retinoids, hyaluronic acid, and even newer amino-acid peptides, stem cells, and skin whiteners. Combinations of several ingredients may offer better efficacy than just one or two. Some cosmeceuticals can irritate your skin when not combined with anti-inflammatory ingredients, so be wary of any irritation that may result from their use.

It is likely some of these active ingredients are already present in your products, and the manufacturer does not refer to them using these terms, selects other terms, or even concocts their own unique term. Confused?

Basically, a "cosmeceutical" is actually a method for those marketing skincare products to imply that there may be ingredients within their products which function better or more successfully than standard ingredients. Of course, the only way to know is to try them and see if they live up to your expectations. And remember to always have realistic expectations.

Don't Panic Over Organic

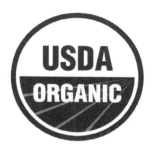

The term "organic" is fortunately better defined than the term "natural." To date, many ingredients are not commercially available certified organic. Why? Because the National Organic Program (NOP) was initiated for the food industry.

Savvy shoppers should learn to distinguish between the various terms before seeking organic products. For crops to be certified organic, they must be grown on land free of pesticides and chemicals for a minimum of three years. *Just three?*

This is interesting because some of those chemicals are not biodegradable. Another criterion is that the agricultural methods must follow National Certified Organic standards to qualify for certification.[22] Different regulatory bodies may have different rules for certification.

There are currently three categories under the National Certified Organic label:

- **100% USDA Certified Organic:** A product labeled as 100% Organic must contain ONLY organically produced ingredients, excluding water and salt.
- **95% Organic:** Organic products must be made with at least 95 percent Certified Organic ingredients (again, excluding water and salt) and may display the USDA Organic seal.
- **Made with Organic Ingredients:** At least 70 percent of the ingredients are organically produced and certified. These products *cannot* display the organic seal.

Even if a producer is certified organic, or utilizing 95 percent certified organic ingredients, they are not required to register them or display the seal. This certification is an expense that not all producers can incur.

Organic is not always necessarily better, as the criteria varies for both organic and natural cosmetics. Some farmers and smaller businesses cannot afford organic certification and we still want to support small and local, right? "All-natural" may be just as good if you can trust the manufacturer. Products with the USDA Organic seal are at least 95 percent organic. This sounds great, right? Well, what if the product yields no visible results? That always stinks!

Finally, wild-crafted ingredients refer to gathering plants in their natural habitat. No chemical additives or manufacturer interference are involved in this process. Often wild-crafting is done sustainably, with a plant being replanted when one is removed or leaving a plant and taking flowers or other elements as needed. Usually respect is shown to endangered species. Now that's great!

Organic is generally defined as "of, related to, or involving the use of food produced with the use of feed or fertilizer of plant or animal origin without the employment of chemically formulated fertilizers, growth stimulants, antibiotics, or pesticides."

As with the term "natural," many companies are using the term "organic" on their labels and in their personal care (beauty) product marketing. If you don't see the USDA organic seal, you will want to use caution. However, products may contain organic ingredients that are not on the USDA organic list, since the criteria was initially established for the food industry. Get to know what ingredients are potentially harmful and avoid them and do your research behind the companies making the claims.

Newer certification bodies are also gaining popularity and all have similar missions in mind to create safer, non-toxic, eco-friendly, and cruelty-free options which means we are on the No Bull path. Yay!

Say No to GMOs!

Genetically Modified Organisms, or GMOs, are plants (for use by humans or animals) that have been modified at the molecular level. Genes are altered to enhance or lessen certain traits. The initial purpose of GMOs was to grow disease-resistant crops and plants that produce more fruit than normal, or don't go bad as quickly after harvest. In health circles, the food forms of GMOs are often referred to as "frankenfoods," which may cause harm to people, animals and the environment. In addition, genetically modified fish and meat, as well as their impact on the environment, are growing health concerns.

Although the long-term effects on humans are still unknown, the FDA has approved more than 40 GMO plants, stating they have completed all federal requirements for commercialization.[23] However, many individuals don't want to put genetically altered food in or on their bodies! If you want to avoid them as well, then *watch out* because some manufacturers are using GMOs in their products and not telling you. For example, modified canola is used to make high levels of lauric acid, an ingredient found in many detergents and soaps.[24] Keep in mind that a lot of plant-based ingredients are used in natural skincare products.

Some common ingredients that may indicate a presence of GMOs include: soybean oil, corn oil, corn flour, proteins from yeast, and lecithin. Avoid them if you can.

To prevent GMOs from getting under your skin there are a few things you can do: know your store, read your labels, and do some research. Then boycott GMOs. Only support companies you know don't use GMO ingredients and who are also in favor of mandatory labeling of all GMO products.

Countries around the world are banning GMOs, yet the US continues to produce over 60 percent of GMO crops and foods. If there is no harm in GMO products then why are huge biotechnology agricultural companies against labeling? There's something wrong here and it's up to us to put a stop to it before it spirals completely out of control and has irreparable consequences!

We should have the right to choose real, not scientifically manipulated food. In doing so, this will also help save the rapidly diminishing bee population which is necessary for a healthy planet. Healthy, natural, unmodified sources are key.

3

The Scoop on Your Skin

Human Skin Anatomy

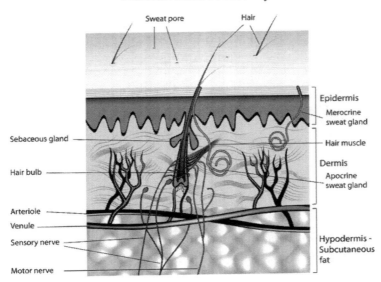

Sweat pore   Hair

Epidermis
Merocrine sweat gland

Sebaceous gland
Hair muscle

Hair bulb
Dermis
Apocrine sweat gland

Arteriole
Venule
Sensory nerve
Hypodermis - Subcutaneous fat
Motor nerve

Getting to Know the Skin You're In

Your skin is the largest organ in the body and is a pathway to your entire body. It is porous and quickly soaks up toxins from the environment and beauty products you use. It's made up of three separate layers called the epidermis, the dermis, and the subcutaneous layer. For the sake of simply understanding the skin you're in, let's break this down layer by layer.

The Epidermis

The epidermis is the thin protective outermost layer of your skin. It offers protection to the deeper layers of the skin, and your organs. This layer consists of keratinocyte cells, which aid in the production of a protective protein called keratin which makes up the structure of the skin, hair, and nails. The epidermis renews itself every month or so and the body is constantly shedding skin cells during this process as new cells arise. The deepest sub-layer of the epidermis known as the basal cell layer, also contains these cells which continually mature, moving towards the surface to create new, fresh skin cells as dead skin cells are shed.

The epidermis is the thinnest on the face and thickest where you need protection from injury, such as the soles of your feet and palms. Melanocyte cells are also contained within the epidermis, and these cells produce a substance that determines skin color called melanin. Melanin is the substance within skin cells that provides some protection against ultraviolet rays. Unfortunately for many, sunburn occurs meaning that the melanin did not have a chance to provide adequate protection. Ever had a tan? Brown spots? You can thank melanin for this.

As you age, epidermal cells do not shed as frequently as they did when you were younger. In addition, the use of common, harsh man-made chemicals and surfactants that strip the skin of its natural oils and protective barrier often result in a dull complexion and lackluster appearance. This is why exfoliating machines, peels, scrubs, fruit acids, retinoids, facials and lasers have become so popular. Everyone wants to get their "glow on" again and maintain their youthful appearance. Exfoliating epidermal cells revitalizes the complexion, although over-exfoliation can actually contribute to inflammation, thinning of the skin, and excessive oil production, which can be detrimental. The key is using natural, gentle products and having more aggressive treatments in moderation.

The Dermis

The dermis is the middle layer of your skin. This layer is much thicker then the epidermis. It contains small blood vessels, nerves, hair follicles, and sweat glands. This is the layer of skin that contains nerve receptors and is responsible for your sense of touch, temperature, pressure, position, and pain. The dermis is held together by protein called collagen. Collagen is the unique compound in your skin that gives it strength, volume, and resilience which contributes to a youthful appearance.

It also plays an important role in wound healing. Collagen is made by cells called fibroblasts and is involved in the production of elastin (a protein that makes your skin flexible). It helps prevent the breakdown of the resistance of your skin to slow pre-mature aging. Think of it this way: collagen and elastin in your skin are like a mattress and box spring, and similar to how the box spring caves and the mattress sags – this ultimately occurs in your skin as you age. The lack of production of these important compounds is a result of hormonal changes, environmental damage from sun exposure and free radicals, inflammation and stress. Avoid and protect against these annoyances every day!

The Subcutaneous Layer

The subcutaneous layer is the deepest layer of your skin. It is attached to the dermis and is held there by collagen and elastin fibers. Composed of a type of cell that accumulates and stores fats called adipocytes, the subcutaneous layer acts as an energy reserve for your skin. It holds fats in the adipocytes until it puts them back into circulation to later be transformed into energy. This is the layer of your skin that participates in burning calories, and actually acts as a thermoregulator, kind of like a thermostat. Pretty cool stuff! The network of collagen fibers and fat cells within this layer protects the body from injury by acting as a shock-absorber.

Because toxins can seep directly into your bloodstream via the epidermis, it's really important to keep these toxic ingredients at the forefront of your mind and avoid them at all costs. Unlike the toxins in foods, which have the opportunity to be filtered before they are stored, the toxins in cosmetics are absorbed directly into your bloodstream and are therefore much more dangerous to cellular health. They can really wreak havoc and launch a toxic assault on your body, at any age. That's why using non-toxic skincare and cosmetic products is so important. Why use products that are designed to keep you looking beautiful when, in reality, they are doing just the opposite and destroying your health?!

Always choose products that do not contain these common toxins. And of course, protect yourself from the sun daily.

The Differing Decades of Aging

My clients seek professional advice and services during various stages of their lives. I continue to see more and more genetic changes and sun damage taking a remarkable toll as we age. The aging process can be fast-tracked if you expose your skin to harsh chemicals, poor diet, and toxic environments. When we are younger, it may be less important because the skin regenerates more often but the problem is that as the skin ages the speed of skin cell regeneration diminishes and the skin thins.

Here's a blow-by-blow account of how the skin ages in each corresponding decade of your life.

The Tricky Teens

Although aging is not yet apparent during these years, other skin problems brought by puberty's hormonal changes or genetics can take place, particularly acne. If left untreated, acne can create scarring and affect self-esteem and other aspects of a teen's life. To counteract this problem, avoid harsh scrubs, sulfates, do not pick the skin and avoid the use of harsh chemicals that can speed up the aging process. Also avoid sun exposure as it will not help acne. Often we think drying out acne is a good thing, when it actually can exacerbate the problem and contribute to aging, excessive oil production, and scarring.

Take Care in Your Twenties

This is often when some basic wear and tear begins to surface. Expression lines begin to show from squinting, smiling, and frowning. Our expression gives us character, so don't fret too much just yet. This breakdown occurs as a result of collagen and elastin depletion. These cushion-like substances are responsible for maintaining the skin's smoothness and suppleness, and this is where our skin's outermost layer is supported like a mattress and box-spring. Don't wait for the day when the damage becomes irreversible and the mattress begins to sag. Start by protecting your skin with nourishing, high-quality ingredients, avoiding excessive sun exposure, eating a healthy unprocessed diet, and toning down the stress.

Get Down and Dirty in Your Thirties

Turn it up a notch during this delightful decade! As the supply of collagen and elastin continues to deplete, wrinkles may evolve during this stage (if not sooner). If the damage is still relatively minimal you can continue to nourish your skin by avoiding harsh environments and select ingredients that expedite the skin's repair and renewal process.

Utilizing antioxidants, fruit acids, natural oils, and omega fatty acids will assist in minimizing the appearance of those flaws and help you prevent further wrinkles from occurring. Keep up with the tips from your 20s, or add them on today!

Don't Fret Your Forties

Dead skin cells are starting to stick around longer. This contributes to a less vibrant appearance and texture. Pigment (dark patches) may become evident and expression lines may appear deeper. Rosacea and/or redness may surface. Don't fret! Quality care and mild exfoliation is needed along with humectants to bind moisture to the skin, as it will start slowing down in terms of oil production. If you are a one of the lucky ones, you may experience oh-so-fun adult acne!

All joking aside, it has its benefits as oil keeps the skin soft and smooth, but acne in your forties is enough to make you frantic. Welcome to perimenopause! Trans-epidermal water loss (TEWL) can fast-track the aging process so keep your skin well hydrated and keep up with the care from your thirties. Aside from committing to a skin care regimen, a diet containing healthy vitamins, essential fatty acids and nutrients for hair, skin, and overall wellness is always essential.

Nothin' but Love for Fifties and Above

If you have survived menopause-induced hormonal imbalances you are doing great! Sunspots, broken capillaries (blood vessels), and wrinkles develop sometimes prior to this time but most commonly during the fifties. If you have been caring for your skin all along, keep it up! Some things are inevitable as genetics play a role in skin and hair aging as well as stress. While you can always undergo surgery, peels, and lasers, holistic options are always less risky. At this time, you may need skin brightening and lightening ingredients, resurfacing fruit acids, and rich, nourishing oils added to your regimen. And remember, it's always a good time to start protecting your skin.

Now that you understand some of the things that occur in the skin during the different stages of your life, let's get a good regimen in place! It's *never* too late to start saving face.

Annoying Acne

Oh, eeeeevil acne! The skin condition that affects the self-esteem of teens and adults alike, and is so frustrating and challenging to combat! Many people waste money on numerous products and have numerous adverse reactions before they find a solution.

What is Acne?

Acne is actually a disease involving the skin. The oil glands produce a liquid called "sebum" that transports dead skin cells through follicles to the skin's surface. When follicles get blocked and sticky skin cells do not shed, the result is acne. Resulting bacteria (propionibacterium acnes) within the blocked follicle cause blemishes and inflammation, and sadly, untreated acne or picking can cause scarring.

Types of Acne

Not all acne conditions are the same, and some are more prone to cause scarring than others. Most people just refer to all kinds of acne as blemishes, but these are the types of acne breakouts most people experience:

1. **Papules:** Tiny pink bumps that are most common.
2. **Whiteheads (Milia):** Visible white bumps appearing just under the skin's surface.
3. **Blackheads:** Visibly dark comedones (clogged pores) on the surface of the skin.
4. **Pustules:** Red, with a pus-filled top.
5. **Cysts:** Often under the skin, common in chin area. Filled with pus and tend to be painful. Most likely to cause scarring.
6. **Nodules:** Large pimples embedded under the skin, but visible on the surface.

Acne can be aggravated by stress, diet, hormonal changes, and a variety of cosmetics, lotions, and hair products that clog the pores. Drying skincare products and sunburns also contribute to acne. Why? Because we often think if we dry up the oil we solve the problem. WRONG! That actually sends a message to the oil glands saying, "protect me" as one of oil's functions is skin protection. Oil naturally protects us from bacteria and environmental invaders while keeping the skin soft and supple. By over-drying the skin via certain products and tanning, we actually exacerbate acne and accelerate aging. Products can also irritate the skin without clearing up acne and might make skin more prone to sunburn because many acne products are skin sensitizers.

Severe acne may require attention from a dermatologist. Harsh medications like Accutane® are prescribed in stubborn cases. This drug is not free from side-effects and is considered highly toxic, so it's a last resort. Other medications may include Spironolactone, antibiotics, and oral contraceptives. Of course, none of these are free from side-effects. Common topical approaches may include salicylic acid-based products, retinoids, fruit acids, anti-inflammatory botanicals and essential oils. In stubborn cases supplementing with oral zinc is often effective as it boosts the immune system, combats pesky bacteria and helps reduce androgen levels. Androgens are annoying hormones that stimulate oil production, which can result in acne; not to mention hair loss or excessive hair growth and other health problems. I find a combination of dietary changes and topical botanical remedies to be highly effective in the treatment of common acne, not to mention safer options. Start with those first.

Milk contains some 60 different hormones (including those androgens) and raises insulin levels dramatically, also affecting the skin and in some cases, contributing to acne. Hormones from dairy products can wreak havoc on your natural hormone balance, so seek organic hormone-free if you desire dairy. Also, as we discuss later, avoiding processed foods that can affect your insulin levels, can help reduce your likelihood of experiencing skin conditions such as acne, rosacea, and pre-mature aging.

Some still think that acne is caused by poor hygiene, but the truth is that washing your face too often can aggravate acne. Not only does frequent washing open up the pustules and spread bacteria, but the skin then produces yet more oil to compensate for the dryness. Intense scrubbing or overuse of mechanical scrubs or machines has the same effect. When you wash your face, start with clean hands, be gentle and use lukewarm water patting your face dry when finished to prevent damage of your skin. To avoid infection, scarring and spread of bacteria, do not pick at your face.

Suffer from adult acne? You are not alone! Dramatic hormonal shifts occur during perimenopause (sometimes earlier) and menopause which may adversely affect the skin. A change in diet, adding a balance of herbal remedies, probiotics and altering your skin care regimen can help reduce and prevent acne at any age!

It is important to find an acne treatment that will not dry out your skin and cause more irritation.

Natural Blemish Busters

Essential Oils

Essential oils offer powerful antibacterial and anti-fungal properties to help fight problem skin conditions. Essential oils of tea tree, grapefruit, bergamot, cedarwood, lavender, ylang ylang, rosemary, lemon, and chamomile are all useful in the treatment of acne. As each oil offers specific properties depending on the type of acne, seek a professional consultation for a recommendation for your specific needs. The essential oils should be diluted in a carrier oil suitable for acne such as hazelnut, hemp, jojoba or grapeseed oil before being applied to the skin.

Fruit Acids (AHAs)

Naturally occurring fruit acids from citrus fruits, grapes, berries, sugar cane and other sources, gently exfoliate skin cells to prevent clogged pores and bacterial growth. These fruit-derived essences also offer brightening properties, and minimize discoloration and scarring.

For a blemish quick-fix simply squeeze the juice of an organic lemon or lime and apply it to affected areas with a cotton swab. Simply rinse and repeat as needed.

Hemp Seed Oil

Hemp seed oil has some of the highest content of EFAs and linoleic acid, rendering its healing and anti-inflammatory properties valuable for resistant acne, psoriasis, and eczema. Super sustainable too!

Licorice Root

Licorice Root is wonderful for evening out the skin's complexion and removing any appearance of discoloration or scarring created by acne. It also protects skin tissue and offers anti-inflammatory properties.

Neem Extract

Because Neem has antibacterial *and* anti-inflammatory properties, it is ideal for treating acne naturally and helping minimize blemishes at the same time.

Purifying Clays

Natural clays such as bentonite, kaolin, and green clay are rich in minerals and vital nutrients. These clays deep cleanse the skin by drawing impurities and absorbing excess oil. You can make a simple mask by adding witch hazel or aloe vera gel to create a spreadable paste. A few drops of tea tree essential oil may be added for stubborn acne. Simply massage onto cleansed damp skin and allow to dry before thoroughly rinsing.

Willow Bark – Natural Salicylic Acid

Willow bark is an excellent natural remedy for acne because it refines skin texture, reduces inflammation, soothes and smoothes skin, and minimizes pore size. Its mild exfoliating action assists in unblocking the follicle to prevent bacteria formation.

Witch Hazel

Witch hazel hydrosol offers natural astringent properties while also reducing inflammation. This ancient herbal remedy for acne makes a wonderful all-natural toner to balance oil and soothe the skin. Avoid the common retail store brands of witch hazel, as the alcohol content will only further irritate acne by stripping the skin. Choose an organic brand whenever possible.

While these are just a few of many effective botanical ingredients, look for these and seek a holistic skin care professional's recommendations to combat acne naturally.

Wicked Rosacea and Redness Relief

Although it may sometimes resemble acne or sensitive skin, rosacea is different. This chronic skin condition is characterized by reddened facial skin with or without the presence of acne lesions. While the symptoms of rosacea tend to be more noticeable in men, women are actually more likely to develop this condition. It often strikes people with fair skin who are between the ages of 30 and 60. Symptoms include redness, a flushed appearance, red nose, and broken capillaries on the face. Sometimes the face has a stinging sensation and the eyes can become watery and bloodshot. In some cases, acne is also present.

Rosacea is a chronic inflammatory skin disorder that is most commonly (but not always) seen in fair skinned individuals. The cause is largely unknown but research suggests that underlying vasomotor instability, cumulative sun damage and a compromised dermal matrix barrier are contributing factors. The presence of the demodex folliculorum mite and the resulting bacterial growth may exacerbate rosacea. Before you get grossed out.... demodex mites are commonly present on the skin. Sorry! They are microscopic and may or may not exacerbate certain skin conditions.

While there is no cure at this time for rosacea and its wicked redness, there are effective ways to treat it. **Consider taking the following steps to minimize the symptoms of rosacea:**

- Minimize your daily stress.
- Lower your intake of spicy foods, alcohol and dairy.
- Reduce activity on very hot days.
- Avoid hot showers and saunas.
- Use sunblock daily and limit your exposure to the sun.
- Avoid skincare products with synthetic fragrance, colors, and dyes.
- Avoid processed foods and eat an anti-inflammatory diet.

- Avoid scrubs and harsh treatments like microdermabrasion.
- Have your hormone levels checked, particularly 25-hydroxy vitamin D.
- Exposure to cold weather, windy days, hot showers or baths and extreme exercise can also exacerbate rosacea.

Many products today are formulated to calm the symptoms of rosacea, but it's trial and error. Make sure to select fragrance-free products that will not irritate your skin.

Recent studies suggest that tea-tree essential oil offers a natural remedy to minimize the presence of bacteria and/or fungus, thus reducing inflammation and redness. Neem seed oil is another natural and effective solution. Many natural plant-derived ingredients such as licorice root, aloe vera, evening primrose oil, panthenol, rose damascena, and calendula (to name just a few) fight reddened, inflamed areas and calm your skin. Seek the guidance of a skin care professional before taking this super sensitive situation into your own hands.

A vitamin D deficiency may also contribute to this skin condition so make sure to have your levels checked and get adequate levels of this super vitamin through diet or supplementation.

When topical remedies and all else fails, laser treatments are often considered. Should you seek this solution, seek a qualified professional. Less is more when it comes to this sensitive skin condition, so just be gentle to your skin and avoid the things that aggravate it.

Dreaded Dark Circles and Aging Eyes

As we age, skin becomes thinner due to the lack of collagen and elastin formation. This may result in wrinkles (crows feet), loss of volume and skin laxity around the eyes. Volume loss in the upper cheeks and under eye area may contribute to a hollow appearance under the eyes, which can lead to noticeable dark circles. Dark circles are not always associated with pigment or melanin as many assume, but instead are often due to leaking capillaries. These leaky blood vessels reveal themselves as a darker color or pigment because they can be seen through the very thin skin of the eyes.

Other causes of dark under eye circles include allergies, medical conditions (thyroid, etc.), heredity, hyperpigmentation, sleep deprivation and environmental exposure.

Good news! -- It is never too late to protect and prevent - here are some tips to help you care for your eye area to prevent and improve dark circles, wrinkles, puffiness and the signs of aging:

- Gently remove eye makeup using a non-drying makeup remover, or pure plant oils such as grapeseed or olive oil.
- Gently tap or lightly apply your products using the ring finger, and *never* drag or pull this fragile skin.
- Avoid dehydrating caffeine and alcohol.
- Limit your sodium intake to help prevent swollen, puffy eyes.
- Drink plenty of water to help flush out harmful substances.
- Elevate your pillows at night to prevent fluid from pooling under the eyes. This will prevent puffy eyes.

- Diets rich in EFAs, vitamin C, and antioxidants can improve the health of your eyes and the skin that surrounds them. These ingredients are also found in high-quality eye care products.
- Get plenty of sleep. Make sure to sleep at least 7 to 9 hours per night and nap as needed.
- Wear UV sunglasses to protect your skin, (and eyes from squinting).
- Use a non-toxic sunblock daily to protect and prevent from future damage. Sun damage also contributes to premature aging of the skin which can lead to wrinkles, pigment issues or fragile capillaries.

If dark circles under your eyes are a constant problem for you, select botanical ingredients such as licorice root, gotu kola, and rose geranium (to name just a few). Natural forms of vitamins A and C are also effective for lightening and brightening, as well as wrinkle reduction.

If you desire a more dramatic approach, cosmetic medical procedures for the eyes include fractionated laser treatments, dermal fillers, blepharoplasty, and fat removal. Use caution here.

Laser procedures are newer technologies which may be useful for wrinkles and leaking capillaries when other methods fail. However, they are not recommended for certain skin tones and you may experience downtime and pain.

Dermal fillers may help minimize the hollow appearance under the eyes and dark circles. However, these "tear trough" injections can be painful and are not free of side effects. In addition, this procedure is not permanent so be sure to research and select a qualified professional or just don't risk it. After all, these are your eyes! It's always best to prevent and protect, and it's never too late. So treat your eyes well!

Awful Age Spots and Pigment Problems

Hyperpigmentation (also referred to as age spots, melasma, pregnancy mask, liver spots, and scarring) often results from excessive sun exposure and trauma to the skin. Patches of skin that are darker in color than the surrounding skin form when an excess of melanin (the brown pigment that produces skin color) forms deposits in the skin. Hyperpigmentation can affect the skin color of people of any race. People with darker Asian, Mediterranean, or African American skin tones are especially prone to this kind of skin disorder. It is also common in women who take birth control pills or experience hormonal changes as a result of pregnancy or other hormonal treatments or imbalances. Additionally, it can be caused by skin diseases, such as acne, that leave dark spots after the condition clears. Prior injuries to the skin, including some surgeries or anything that results in inflammation may lead to this type of scarring. Previous sun damage is a VERY common culprit that not only causes age spots but also dramatically accelerates aging.

Now how do you treat this common and usually harmless skin condition? Many prescription creams used to lighten the skin contain hydroquinone, but I don't recommend that toxic ingredient. Retinoid products have also long been used as a treatment for pigmentation. While they are effective, they often have side effects. Fortunately, today we have natural alternatives and ingredients to lighten and fade darkened skin patches by slowing the production of melanin. In turn, those pesky dark spots gradually fade to match normal skin coloration.

Natural treatment ingredients include licorice root, vitamin C, neem, niacinamide (vitamin B3), botanical extracts such as willow bark, fruit acids, rosehip seed oil and more. Laser treatments are also effective but often require numerous treatments and carry negative side effects including but not limited to, pain, hypopigmentation, and possible recurrence.

No matter how you choose to treat these darkened areas, you must use a sunblock daily. Melanin in the skin has memory, and even the smallest amount of sun exposure can reproduce the dark spot you are trying to erase. Another benefit to using a physical sunblock (mineral) is that you will also prevent premature wrinkling and sagging of the skin as well. Just make sure to use a reputable brand. Use caution to protect your skin and you will retard the aging process while avoiding sun damage and hyperpigmentation, age spots, possible cancers, and even wrinkles!

Hypopigmentation, on the other hand, is a loss of pigment (or melanin) in the skin. These white or light colored patches are much more difficult to treat then hyperpigmentation. However, this discoloration is also often a result of inflammation, scars and skin damage. As medical conditions and other factors may contribute to this condition, seek the opinion of a medical professional and do your best to keep inflammation at bay. Steroid use, auto-immune disorders and other factors may also result in this loss of pigment.

You Can't Win with Dry Skin

Dry skin may present itself as flaky, dull or simply lackluster. But did you know that dry skin is actually more prone to injury, aging, and even scarring? Proper skin hydration is essential to prevent long-term damage. To understand why your skin may undergo such changes, a phenomenon known as trans-epidermal water loss (TEWL) is important to understand.

TEWL pertains to the measurement of the water, which goes from inside the body to the surrounding atmosphere via the epidermal (outer) layer of your skin. Increased TEWL is *not* ideal. TEWL can increase due to change of season, hormonal changes or even the climate you live in. Damaging sunburns and irritating or drying ingredients can also boost TEWL.

Having oily skin does not mean you won't fall victim to TEWL at some point. Flying long distances or not drinking enough water will also deplete your skins moisture levels. Be sure to drink 8-10 glasses of filtered or reverse osmosis water daily. You can also obtain water, along with other vital nutrients, from fruits and vegetables such as cucumbers, watermelon or celery. But the good news is, there are ways to prevent TEWL and win the fight against dry, lackluster skin!

Hooray for Humectants!

When applied to the skin, humectants plump, hydrate the skin and help to prevent TEWL, dryness and accelerated aging. These substances absorb water from the air and hold moisture in the skin.

91

They are effective at softening and minimizing flaky, dry, dull skin. Hyaluronic acid, for example, can hold up to 1,000 times its weight in water, rendering it one of the best weapons against dehydration and aging. Some take this in supplement form to lubricate joints and alleviate pain. An alternative to hyaluronic acid is vegetable glycerin, which also offers humectant properties, kills bacteria, and reduces inflammation. These super ingredients lock in moisture and prevent TEWL without clogging pores. Hooray!

Exfoliation

During the aging process skin cells accumulate and stick around longer, so exfoliation of these sluggish surface dwellers may become necessary. Removal of these uppermost dead skin cells will minimize flaking, promote a healthy glow and enable your humectant-filled products to penetrate more effectively. Just be careful not to "over-exfoliate," and refer to my section on scrubs and scrapers to learn more. Always seek a professionals advice before using harsh exfoliants, abrasive ingredients or devices. You may also consider adding mild fruit-acids and gentle enzymes to your regimen, which gently dissolve skin cells often with little to no irritation.

These types of ingredients along with cell-protecting antioxidants, omega fatty acids, humectants and botanical extracts are some of the best combinations to win the war against dry skin and premature aging. To achieve optimum results, eat well, cut out unhealthy sodas, artificial sweeteners, high-fructose corn syrup, hydrogenated oils, processed sugars, GMOs, dairy and gluten.

Always remember, what goes in must come out. Since your skin is one of the largest organs (and a detoxification organ), you might find it coming out on the surface of your skin.

The Fight Against Free Radicals

Whether you are young or old, unwelcome changes may occur resulting in wrinkles and dry, dull skin. Environmental factors such as free radical damage just may be the culprit.

Free radicals are unstable molecules that scavenge and attack healthy cells. While their production occurs inside the body, they also result from UVA (sun damage), pollution, smoking, toxic chemicals, alcoholic beverages, and unhealthy diet. The cellular damage caused by free radicals is what significantly contributes to aging.

If free radicals are in abundance, then your cells are subjected to more severe damage, which can fast track aging, damage tissues, and even result in diseases. Think of a peeled apple that has been untouched for a couple of minutes. From its crisp state, the fruit starts to turn brown (oxidize) and quickly turn unpleasant. This is caused by free radicals. But if you squeeze just a touch of lemon juice on those apples, they stay fresh and crisp, and the browning reaction does not occur. Pretty cool, right?

The good news is that there is a lemon-juice solution to ward off free radical damage in your skin as well: antioxidants. Antioxidants are the "good guys" because they provide your body with ample oxygen molecules. If there is a plentiful supply of these molecules, your body's defense mechanism is strengthened and free radicals can actually be deactivated. Antioxidants come in the form of vitamins, minerals, and other nutrients. These molecules strengthen the enzymes that regenerate your body's damaged cellular tissue and even DNA.

Amazing Antioxidants

To protect against free radical damage, antioxidants are a must! Some foods are excellent sources of antioxidants, including pomegranate, lemons, grapes, blueberries, acai berries, goji berries, garlic, mushrooms, carotenes, extra virgin olive oil, and even dark (raw/unprocessed) chocolate! Green tea, and red tea (rooibos) are also rich sources of antioxidants. It's advisable to get as many antioxidants from food sources as you can, and consult your physician before taking supplements if you are unsure about them. Antioxidants (both internally and externally) are essential for anti-aging as they combat free radical damage and help renew skin from past cellular injury, while also minimizing lines, wrinkles, and more.

With naturally-derived vitamins like these, a combination of free-radical fighting products, and proper diet can deliver amazing results including cell regeneration, protection from environmental stressors and may even significantly minimize lines, wrinkles, and age spots! It's never too late to put up a fight against free radicals.

Inflammation Nation

Inflammation Ages You – Boooo!

At some point in your life, you will awake to observe and feel not-so-welcome changes in your body. But do you know that some of the wrinkles and dreaded diseases are not actually by-products of natural aging? Researchers now know a big part of the aging process actually results from inflammation.

As its name suggests, an inflammatory process triggers increased blood flow to the tissue, which in turn leads to swelling and pain. Next time you say "ouch," think about this biochemical process, which is an automatic response from your immune system each time it encounters a harmful stimulus. Although you might think that inflammation is an essential part of life, it can occur even in the absence of harm. Your body can become paranoid!

This paranoia can pave way for destructive diseases like arthritis, asthma, allergies, diabetes, lupus, skin diseases, psoriasis and a lot more. Once your immune system becomes weakened, it loses the ability to determine when to use or not use its inflammatory response.

Aging and inflammation go hand in hand because the latter's presence causes free radical damage to the cells. Not only can your skin become collateral damage, but your whole body as well! Avoid products that cause inflammation and, of course, try to minimize sun damage, as the change in pigmentation is a result of inflammation and it ages you. It also causes those pesky age spots, and may increase your risk of developing cancer too.

Inhibiting inflammatory responses can be achieved by maintaining a healthy diet. Avoidance of pro-inflammatory substances like trans-fats, sweets and fried food has been proven helpful. One of the wonders of omega-3 essential fatty acids is their anti-inflammatory ability. As antioxidants neutralize free radicals, omega-3's calm the inflammation. Just make sure to balance them with omega-6 fatty acids. Follow these tips and minimize stress to protect your skin and prevent inflammatory aging.

4

Beauty Gone Wild

Fillers, Drillers and Lasers OH MY!

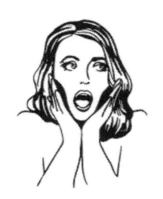 Men and women are going gaga over dermatological treatments that offer noticeable results in a furious flash. Sure, it's nice to see results in less than five sessions or so. Like a magic wand, fillers, lasers, and botulinum toxin injections are some of the industry's common procedures that demonstrate great efficacy in treating numerous skin problems like pimples, scarring, wrinkles, uneven skin tone, and age spots.

If you are tempted to try one of these procedures you should first know that the big price tag might also be a risky one. If want to have a wrinkle-free (and possibly frozen or freakish appearing) face, these are super fast options. Just make certain you have a true industry specialist treating you and not any Joe Shmoe because trust me, there are plenty of so-called specialists reaping the cash benefits of this cosmetic business. So proceed with caution.

Let's Compare Some Popular Treatments:

Injectable fillers are available under brand names such as Restylene®, Juvederm®, Radiesse®, Perlane®, and Belotero® (the list goes on and on). Hyaluronic acid based fillers are commonly used for plumping and filling areas including the cheekbones, lips, nasolabial folds and even hollows in the under eye area. They are longer lasting than botulinum toxin (Botox®, etc.), and can be used in areas of the face where botulinum toxin is contraindicated. They are used to plump and firm without the need for a facelift. The reduction of collagen and elastin as we age results in sagging skin, loose skin, thinner skin and lips, and nasolabial folds (also known as marionette lines). These funky gel substances literally fill facial lines, add facial contours and even plump the lips. When you decide to have a filler treatment, a clear gel made of hyaluronic acid will commonly be injected into your skin or lips. These treatments are not free of side effects.

Bruising appears to be the most common annoyance, which means you may not be out socializing for a good few days after, so seek the most qualified injector possible. Results are temporary, so be prepared to pay for it one to two times per year if you are satisfied with the results and do not mind the pain.

There are longer-lasting filler options and new brand names available often, but I would recommend ensuring you are pleased first before going with a more permanent option. Lumps and bumps may result, which are certainly not ideal if permanent.

Laser procedures on the other hand, offer popular treatments to minimize wrinkles and age spots, may improve skin texture, diminish acne scars, reduce hair growth, and more. There are many types of lasers available for a variety of skin conditions and hair removal.

There are IPL (intense pulsed light), hair removal lasers and the newer fractional lasers for full skin resurfacing along with many other laser technologies. Now just remember these don't always come without risk. Side effects may include too much or too little pigmentation, scarring, infection and more. You must also consistently protect the treated areas from sun exposure and make sure to follow the physician's recommendations to avoid infection for optimal results. Other risks can include, but are not limited to: temporary redness, downtime, flaking, and peeling. In addition, most lasers require multiple treatments, some as many as six or more for lasting results. Often, more treatments are needed for hair removal so be cautious when seeking laser treatment, because it is not always permanent. Because of the hormone's role in hair production, it is a challenge to permanently remove the hair (particularly in the facial area). Phrases like "permanent reduction" are often used. Watch out for that type of play on words!

Are Lasers for You?

In most cases, laser treatments are not recommended for Asian, Mediterranean or darker skin types, including African American. However, a patch test may be performed. The general rule is: the fairer the skin, the better the candidate. This is because the laser light is attracted to darker pigments and imposes a risk of burning or discoloring the skin, so a lower setting is required. Alternatives at a lesser cost may include home care with active ingredients or a series of professional peel treatments.

Botox®: Miracle or Mirage?

Botox® (and other brands of botulinum toxin) injections are presently the most popular "quick fix" for wrinkles. There are additional options under various brand names to date, but all offer the same potential risks and side effects. These are pharmaceutical drugs developed from botulinum toxin. So, is this something you want to inject into your face for a quick fix? If your answer is yes, then you should know how this popular remedy works, and consider the possible side effects.

The botulinum toxin acts by blocking neurotransmitters to the muscle, reducing or eliminating muscular contractions. The side effect of this facial muscle paralysis is the reduction of movement and also wrinkling in that particular area. Since these muscles are now partially paralyzed, the wrinkles can no longer form. Areas that are not treated with botulinum toxin will not be affected. Botulinum toxin injections are not recommended for certain areas in order to avoid inhibiting important muscular actions that should not be interfered with, such as the mouth area. Primary sites for these injections are around the eyes or forehead as loss of muscular action has been said not to cause functional problems in these areas. If botulinum toxin is injected into the wrong group of muscles, adverse effects like muscle weakness, uneven brows, droopy eyelids, voice hoarseness, and blurry vision can result. That's something serious to consider. Also, the toxins can easily merge into other areas so other side effects may result. Fortunately, this is reversible in most cases but is clearly not ideal. Of course, you should know that not all errors are the result of the product but also technician technique, so using caution in selecting a qualified technician is essential!

The effects of these injections last several months, which is good if you are satisfied with the result, but bad if you cannot afford to keep up the maintenance. Subsequent treatments will be required to prevent recurrence of wrinkles. In some cases, the body develops antibodies to the toxin that reduce its effectiveness, and certain medicines are also said to have the same result. This is a treatment that some people become resistant to, requiring additional expenses and visits.

Side effects of injections most commonly include bruising and swelling at the injection site, headaches, rashes, and for some people, flu-like symptoms. *The list goes on!* And well, the name has the word "toxin" right there in your face, so if that is all okay with you, then you should research it further and seek a qualified injector. While a non-invasive approach to anti-aging is always preferred, the desire for a "quick fix" understandably appeals to many, and there are options galore!

Do Scrubs + Scrapers = Time Erasers?

Microdermabrasion

Another popular beauty treatment that has been buzzing for awhile is microdermabrasion. In this procedure, crystals are sprayed onto your skin to exfoliate or peel the external layers. Alternatively, a diamond tip wand is used to abrade the skin without the use of messy crystals. Some people end up inhaling the powder during the procedure and experience a myriad of reactions as a result, making the diamond tip wand a safer option. The same end result occurs despite the fancy names and type of treatment wand used.

Many people believe that microdermabrasion offers results including smoother skin, reduced pimple scars and age spots, and a renewed complexion. Microdermabrasion is a quick procedure, and may be effective for some skin conditions (if performed properly), but it also can lead to broken capillaries (blood vessels), redness, exacerbate rosacea and create ugly patches if the pressure is too aggressive or the individual's skin is highly sensitive. Smaller versions of these popular systems are also available for at-home use. These machines however, may be riskier. The quality is often inferior and applying incorrect pressure can cause more harm than good.

Make sure a true professional treats you if you want to indulge. Do not expect this to be a "magic wand" though. While microdermabrasion is effective at smoothing the skin and minimizing imperfections a series of treatments often produces better results than just one. It is also not a good option for those with fragile and sensitive skin types. If you are one of these folks, you may need to select a less abrasive alternative. There are so many manufacturers of these systems out there, and the popularity of microdermabrasion can make it difficult to know if what you're getting is really a quality treatment.

Scrub and Device Advice

Over-the-counter products such as scrubs, rotating mechanical devices, and mild peels are additional alternatives to exfoliate and renew the skin. But do they really work? The skin on the body is thicker and less fragile, so scrubs are a nice option to smooth away flaky old skin cells. You can even make your own body scrub with vegetable oils from your cupboard by combining them with finely ground cane sugar or ground oats. Easy stuff! However, caution should be used when applying scrubs to facial skin as it is much more delicate and comprised of fragile capillaries which can leak if too much pressure, abrasive materials or rotating devices are applied. Aggressive scrubbing and overuse of devices can cause microscopic scarring and pinpoint bleeding. The mildest of pressure should be used when working on the face, throat, and décolleté areas.

The popularity of home skincare devices has been of great concern to me as an aesthetician because: a) they can exacerbate conditions of acne or rosacea; b) they are not often sterilized regularly; and c) if overused, they can cause inflammation, which in turn equals aging. Less is more when you are treating your skin at home. It's better to err on the side of caution.

Alternatively, consider a professional facial. Facials offer a multitude of benefits for the skin. When performed by an experienced professional, facials can improve skin tone, texture and radiance while minimizing imperfections. A facial will generally include the use of an exfoliant, enzyme or mild peeling for your skin type to remove sluggish surface skin cells and refine skin texture. Additional steps will be taken to deep clean pores, balance sebum (oil) production, and firm and tone the skin. The facial massage increases circulation, promotes collagen and flushes impurities (toxins) from the skin. Ask your specialist in advance what type of products he/she uses to avoid any irritating or toxic ingredients.

To maintain the benefits of any procedure, a healthy diet, drinking plenty of water, and the use of quality home care products are essential.

Massage: Massaging the skin promotes tissue regeneration, relaxes overused muscles, enhances immunity by stimulating lymphatic drainage (the body's natural purification and defense system), increases circulation, promotes a healthy glow and enhances collagen production. When applying your skincare products, massage with upward and outward motions, using gentle but firm pressure while lifting up the skin. Apply gentle pressure around the eyes, using your ring finger, starting from the outside working inwards. Make sure not to neglect the jawline, neck and décolleté. For the body or scalp, use a fruit or vegetable-derived oil such as grapeseed, coconut or olive oil and don't be afraid to massage your skin, scalp and body, as the benefits are beautifying! Consider consulting with a skin care professional to learn more massage techniques.

The Deal on Peels

Another trendy procedure is the "lunchtime" or chemical peel. These peels may include AHA (alpha hydroxy fruit acids), salicylic acid (beta hydroxy for acne), TCA (trichloracetic acid), and many more.

A variety of chemical peels exfoliate the skin to minimize imperfections, age spots, acne, wrinkles, and more. However, not all peels are the same. The lunchtime peels generally refer to glycolic acid or AHA (alpha hydroxy acid) peels and are milder, with little to no downtime.

Alpha hydroxy acids refer to the naturally occurring acids derived from lemons, oranges, sugar cane, sugar maple, bilberries, grapes, and more. These natural derivatives gently dissolve the sluggish uppermost skin cell layers to generate new cell formation and minimize facial flaws. As we age, skin cells do not shed as rapidly as when we are younger. As a result you may experience a dull, tired, and lackluster complexion. Glycolic acid may be derived from sugar cane (or synthesized in a lab), and has the smallest molecular structure of all of the AHA's. It enhances collagen and elastin production while encouraging newer healthier cell production and minimizing imperfections. These peels often vary in pH and may cause mild stinging or temporary redness. A test patch is recommended for highly sensitive individuals. Results may not be dramatic from these milder peels, but they are generally a safe and effective way to improve the texture of the skin and promote a healthy glow. Who doesn't want to get their glow on?

Beta Hydroxy Acid peels such as salicylic acid are utilized to treat and control acne, regulate sebum (oil) excretion, and remove dead skin cells. These are fairly gentle peels and best indicated in the treatment of acne.

Enzyme peels are generally mild and gently exfoliate the skin to reveal a smoother texture and improved radiance. These peels are ideal for very sensitive skin and are my kind of peel. Natural fruit enzyme peels may include pumpkin, pineapple, cherry, and even banana. They often smell just as yummy as they feel.

Jessner's peel is a combination of salicylic acid, resorcinol, and lactic acid. This peel was pioneered by Dr. Jessner, a dermatologist who developed the peel to remove the superficial layers of skin thus minimizing imperfections, scarring, and even acne.

TCA (Trichloroacetic acid) peels are more aggressive and intended to minimize hyperpigmentation, deeper lines, and scars. TCA can be used in varying strengths and is most commonly used for medium depth peeling. A qualified skin specialist or physician should administer these peels. Again, a patch test is recommended. Downtime commonly occurs from this type of peeling and great care of your skin both pre and post-procedure is essential.

Phenol peels are the "Big Kahuna" of peels. This super aggressive chemical peel is reserved for those with very deep lines, coarsely wrinkled skin, deep scars and/or uneven pigment. Phenol peels are strictly for extreme cases and not without risk, as you can imagine. This was the classic chemical peel. Today, in many cases, lasers are used as a chemical-free alternative.

Other peeling methods are often condition-specific and new ones surface regularly. Remember, no matter what you pay or how companies claim something is "tried and tested," this does not guarantee that *you* won't experience unwanted side effects. Hundreds of reports each year state that patients experience swelling, reddening, prolonged stinging, and darkening of treated areas. *Do your homework, or just don't do it.*

Also, if you have any treatment too often, you only make the skin's layers thinner, making it oh-so-vulnerable to damage from the sun and environment. Remember to always use your sunblock.

Why Toy with Retinoids?

Retinoids are one of the commonly-found ingredients in beauty products that claim to battle aging. Retinoids are a class of chemical compounds related to vitamin A. Retinol and retinoic acid are both types of retinoids. Retinoids require a prescription whereas retinols are generally sold over the counter. Retinols convert to retinoic acid within our bodies but this process is slower.

What Should You Know About Retinoids?

Initially, retinoids were developed to treat resistant acne. It was later discovered that retinoids also assist in combating premature signs of aging, particularly wrinkles. Many product manufacturers claim that retinoids improve the elasticity of the skin by boosting the production of elastin and collagen. They assert that retinoids work within, to repair past damage and rejuvenate skin texture, tone, and elasticity while also reducing the appearance of sun spots, blemishes, and pigment problems. It is believed that instead of working on just the skin's outside layers, retinoids contain an antioxidant component that acts to combat free radicals. While I do emphasize that free radicals and inflammation are one of the leading causes of aging and cellular injury, this ingredient should be avoided unless you intend to take special care of your skin.

Are Retinoids for You?

Some users may experience a dull, flaky, sensitive or reddened appearance to their skin. Recent studies also reveal this ingredient may be carcinogenic.[25] *What?!* Here is why: Retinoids are regarded for their ability to remove dead cells, but as a result of this exfoliating property, the skin becomes more vulnerable to sunlight. Continuous use of retinoid products can thin your skin and make you more vulnerable to sun damage, which can contribute to skin cancer. Dermatologists recommend the usage of retinoids at night to avoid sun exposure as well as to take advantage of its therapeutic properties, as your skin cells regenerate during the sleep cycle.

To minimize sensitivity, your physician may suggest that you initially apply retinoid creams every other day or every third day until your skin becomes acclimated. Another option I suggest to my retinoid-using clients is to apply it over a light layer of cream, which will reduce the penetration rate. You will also want to keep your skin well hydrated and stay protected from sun, heat, cold, and even the heat of a hair dryer directed at the face. Sounds complicated, eh?

If you're pregnant or currently breastfeeding, retinoids should be avoided. If you suffer from hormonal acne throughout your pregnancy, you should seek advice from a medical professional.

So, Do Over-The-Counter Retinols Deliver?

Skin care counters are filled with products that claim to harness the power of retinol (which comes in many forms). Despite studies that support the efficacy of retinols, not all dosages will work for everybody. While you may experience fewer side effects than in prescription form, you may not experience the same benefits. As we all have varied skin types and imperfections we seek to improve, it will always be best to consult with an expert. This is to ensure that your skin will not react harshly from sensitizing ingredients, and that you choose the right product for your skin type.

Are There Alternatives to Retinoids?

Retinoids definitely play a notable role in the anti-aging industry and if used accordingly, can provide noticeable results. But are the possible side effects worth it? The good news is there are cutting-edge botanical products that offer similar results via natural sources. Ingredients that contain beta-carotene, (found in red, yellow, orange fruits and vegetables), convert to vitamin A within the skin if your body needs it, otherwise it roams around to find and squelch damaging free radicals. Natural topical sources of beta carotene include carrot seed oil, sea buckthorn berry, rosehip seed oil, blue-green algae, and more.

If you should opt to try a retinol or retinoid product, make sure to select one that combines soothing botanical anti-inflammatory agents to combat any irritation. You can include vitamin A from natural sources in both your diet and skincare products to experience the benefits with less risk.

Hair Loss Hazards

There are a variety of self-proclaimed "miracle cures" on the market that claim to turn thinning hair into a thick mane. Is thin-to-thick hair really possible? Are these products too good to be true or just more bogus beauty claims?

Some hair loss sufferers are desperate but cannot purchase these so-called miracles because of the hefty price tags. Others have tried them but discovered they must use them for life to maintain the results (if they even work). You may wonder why they work for some but not others. It seems unfair. To know which hair loss remedies will work for you, you must first determine the cause of your hair loss.

Hair loss can result from normal aging, hormonal changes, stress, post-partum hormonal flux, or from thyroid or autoimmune diseases. A blood test is recommended to find out if any of these conditions are the culprit. Genetics, dermatitis, and even allergies may also play a role in hair loss, and so can beauty products. It is difficult to treat hair loss without first ruling out medical conditions. Vitamin and mineral deficiencies can also contribute to hair loss and excessive shedding, including sparse lashes and brows.

Hair loss products are available in the form of supplements or topical formulations. The newer topical formulas are similar to the eyelash conditioners and may contain vitamins, amino-acid peptides, and botanicals to nourish hair follicles. Some companies claim speedy results. However, that may not necessarily be what everyone experiences. So for people suffering from hair loss, if it works it may be good! Some users complain of sticky textures and inflated price tags, and then what happens if you stop using them? In most cases, the hair just resorts to its prior condition.

Biotin, a water-soluble B-vitamin, is useful for hair loss in the case of deficiency, when 5 mg is taken daily. Having your iron and D3 (hydroxy 25) levels checked might also detect a deficiency. Eating foods rich in these nutrients along with omega fatty acids will help support healthier hair and scalp to combat hair loss naturally.

Minoxidil is sold under the brand name Rogaine® and once stood alone as the leader in hair loss products with a proven efficacy. Potential side effects of using Minoxidil include skin irritation, contact dermatitis, dry or flaking scalp and itching. These side effects increase for people with sensitive skin. It is not recommended for pregnant or nursing women or for people using other topical medications. It is also potentially toxic to humans and pets, so use with caution. Specialists claim that minoxidil for women is ineffective and that the men's formulation is a better choice. This topical treatment often grows fine vellus hairs (aka "baby hairs") which often disappoint. This product must also be used for life or you may just lose your re-growth.

Men have the option of the oral drug finasteride, sold under the brand name Propecia®. This drug cannot even be handled by women due to possible toxic effects. However, in many cases men are able to maintain a full head of hair using this drug. As the causes of female and male hair loss vary, unfortunately the treatments vary as well.

Many hair thickening products can be super slimy and create a residue, making the hair appear even thinner. There are other options including laser combs and caps, which are extremely pricey but can the science behind them back up their lofty claims? The combs are a bit frustrating to use, making the costly cap more appealing, but certainly not fun.

Avoid tight ponytails, sulfate shampoos, ammonia hair color (or all hair dye if possible) and relaxers. P-Phenylenediamine (PPD) is a chemical substance widely used in hair dye. It may cause dermatitis and allergic reactions affecting the scalp and hair, and its cumulative effects are potentially toxic. Also avoid straightening procedures, toxic Brazilian blowouts (whew are these treatments scary) and permanent waves. While henna may be advertised as natural, it often contains metallic elements that are best avoided if you suffer from hair loss. Also dispose of leave-in hair products, as they may clog the follicles/pores of your scalp.

Doing an apple cider vinegar rinse on occasion will remove the toxic buildup of film on the scalp, freeing the follicles to produce hair more effectively. It will also impart beautiful shine to the hair. Rosemary and peppermint have also been proven effective in clearing the scalp of debris and stimulating the follicle to produce new growth. This is why you see an abundance of "rosemary mint" products on the market. However, these ingredients appear to work better if massaged into the scalp vs. immediately washed off.

If hair loss is a problem for you, see a physician to rule out medical conditions and make sure to use non-toxic hair care products with gentle ingredients and pure essential oils. I also recommend inverted yoga postures as they increase circulation to the scalp. Thin or sparse hair can be aided with a number of options, so consider them all before making a decision. You don't have to expose yourself to pricey products that are most likely too good to be true to get the results you desire.

Lash and Brow Lowdown

So why do my eyelashes and eyebrows seem so sparse anyway?

Unfortunately, hair follicles deteriorate over time as a result of hormone changes, natural aging, and other factors. Because of this deterioration, hair including that on the eyebrows, scalp, and eyelashes tends to turn brittle and fall out easily. This hair falls out even more when we use products like eyelash curlers, extensions, and mascara frequently. Also, some people just genetically have thinner hair.

As with hair loss, medical issues such as thyroid conditions or nutritional deficiencies can affect how thick, lush or sparse your brows and lashes appear, so never neglect seeking medical attention with any hair loss, whether it is a sudden change or a gradual loss.

Eyelash products that promise fuller, longer lashes seem to be in abundance these days. But how do we know which ones really work and which are any potentially harmful? Some of these products contain prostaglandin analogs (hormone-like substances) along with botanicals and peptides. Some of these active ingredients contribute to the product's efficacy, but may also have unwanted side effects.

There are options via prescription, over the counter, and in beauty salons for products promising thicker, longer, more lush lashes (and even hair). Some labels indicate possible side effects such as change in eye color or pigment of the skin it comes in contact with, as well as growing hair in related areas. Some "hormone-like" ingredients can enter the bloodstream and act as endocrine disruptors. But as they are newer to the market, the data is limited here.

Remember if these products work for you, you will need to use them for life to maintain the benefits, so be sure to select a cost-effective, safe solution for your needs that you can use long term.

The solution to stopping the deterioration and loss of eyelashes may take some trial and error. Essential fatty acids and vitamins such as biotin, as recommended for scalp hair, are also useful for lashes and brows. Eyelashes can be regrown in many cases, but make sure you are not damaging the follicles even more by using harmful products. Most importantly, make sure to seek medical advice to ensure that you are not ignoring an underlying health condition.

Luscious Lip Tips

If you have thinner looking lips, it could be for a number of reasons. Genetics plays the largest role, along with natural aging, but too much sun exposure can also thin out the lips by breaking down the elastin and collagen fibers. Cigarette smoking destroys collagen production, contributing to aging lips as well. The skin of the lips, as well as around them is quite thin, fragile, and prone to fine lines and wrinkles, so use caution when selecting your lip products. You will want to protect your lips from the sun and nourish them with natural oils that provide antioxidant protection and essential nutrients.

Vertical lip lines above the lips may also result of from drinking with straws and too much puckering. And of course, cigarette smoking. Try not to make funny faces, sip from straws, smoke or smooch all day long if you want to avoid those annoying lip lines.

Hydrating and protecting the lips is essential to prevent a dry, cracked appearance. So, to avoid the pesky vertical lines that present themselves with age, don't assume a lip plumper is the solution. Prevention is the best remedy.

So What is a Lip Plumper?

A lip plumper usually comes in a gloss form, or sometimes even has a gel-like or cream consistency. The ingredients may vary, but usually the result is fuller looking lips.

Some lip plumpers also promote skin regeneration and mildly

exfoliate, giving lips a smoother feeling. Ideally, they help to retain moisture, which results in a firmer and fuller feel. If you are expecting a miracle though, don't hold your breath. Results are often temporary, though some products are more effective than others.

You should stop using a product if you experience intense burning sensations, skin discoloration, redness around the lips or damaged skin. When you apply a lip plumper, you may feel a tingle and sometimes the feeling is cooling. When the plumper makes your lips feel very hot and painful, that usually means you are experiencing a negative reaction to the product and should seek one that is better for your lips.

Some folks prefer the fast fix of injectable fillers, which are longer-lasting but also have their share of side effects, not to mention an awful appearance if not done by a real pro.

Not all lip plumpers are bad, yet there is not enough research as to whether using a plumping gloss too much can actually harm the lips. If you do decide to use a lip plumper, use it sparingly and preferably not every day.

In summary, avoiding the sun, smoking, crappy chemical-filled lipsticks, and puckering can help maintain the fragile skin of the lips and areas surrounding them. Applying all-natural lip products daily and/or pure natural oils will also keep your lips soft, luscious and supple, and may help prevent vertical lip lines.

5

Crap-Free Living and Lifestyle

Multi-Purpose Cabinet Keepers

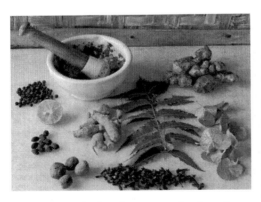 Here are several natural, non-toxic "keepers" that you should always have within arm's reach. You already raided your cabinet, so now you get to refill it with the following fantastic dual-purpose goodies for uses around the house and also for overall wellness. As with anything, read the labels and make sure you purchase your products from a reputable source.

Acai Berry

Acai berry offers antibacterial, anti-inflammatory, and antioxidant properties. Jam-packed with EFAs (essential fatty acids), phytonutrients, vitamins, antioxidants, minerals, and enzymes, Acai is an anti-aging powerhouse! You can use this berry in powder or liquid form for smoothies, or as a supplement to boost antioxidant health. Acai berry tea will also help ward off free radicals and offer protection from the inside out!

Aloe Vera

Aloe vera is great for skin cell regeneration. This super hydrator offers numerous vitamins and nutrients for cellular repair and renewal. Aloe is a soothing solution for skin irritation, sunburn, eczema, and a variety of skin conditions.

I like to keep a few of these plants around the house. Simply cut off a leaf, peel back the skin, and apply the gel from the leaves to irritated areas and experience the soothing relief of aloe. Just make sure not to get it on your clothing. Aloe vera also contains numerous vitamins that benefit internal health. Try squeezing some of the fresh juice or gel into smoothies.

Apple Cider Vinegar

Apple cider vinegar (or ACV) is one of my favorite household staples. A tablespoon of ACV in a cup of cold water makes a wonderful hair rinse after shampooing to impart shine and increase volume. Re-purpose an old bottle and store this blend to use a few times a week or as needed.

Added to water, ACV naturally detoxifies and purifies the liver. This may be useful for healthy immunity and to promote vibrant skin. For weight maintenance (and even weight loss), research suggests 2 tablespoons added to a large glass of water may be effective.

Add a ½ cup of ACV to 1 cup of water, and keep this in a spray bottle to clean and disinfect glass, kitchen surfaces, microwaves, windows, and toilets. This ancient remedy is great for just about everything. ACV is a natural bug repellant, blemish treatment (diluted), house cleaner, purifier, and much more! Choose an organic brand and give it a whirl. It's kinda stinky, but in a good way.

Argan Oil

Packed full of vitamin E and omega fatty acids, argan oil is widely used for cosmetic purposes as well as internally as it is edible. Topically, this antioxidant-rich oil moisturizes the skin and hair.

Don't be fooled though. The beauty industry has adulterated this precious oil and slapped the name on labels everywhere, yet it is often diluted with chemical offenders. Pure organic argan oil is your best bet. It is a healthy gourmet cooking oil, but be sure to avoid high heat. Its faint nutty flavor is perfect for homemade salad dressings and sautéing mushrooms.

Avocado

Rich in essential fatty acids, minerals, and vitamins, avocado oil promotes the skin's natural ability to protect itself as well as soothes inflammation and irritation. Avocado is a great source of phytonutrients and antioxidants. Orally, this superfood is great for healthy skin, nails, and hair. And you can mash an avocado and apply it as a conditioning hair or facial mask!

Bananas

Bananas are rich in vitamins A, E, C, and B along with minerals and amino acids which help promote healthy skin and hair. An abundant source of potassium, natural oils, and enzymes, this fruit is an excellent emollient and superfood.

Topically, a combination of mashed banana and olive oil offers a quick nourishing facial mask. The addition of some ground oats will sooth irritated skin. Treat your hair to an all-natural conditioning treatment by combining mashed avocado, banana, and some coconut oil.

As a food source, if you are concerned about the carb content, you can simply choose baby bananas or reduce your portion size. The vitamins and nutrients bountiful in bananas may help reduce blood pressure and promote muscle maintenance in addition to alleviating bloating. Add a banana to your smoothies for texture, flavor, fiber, and a great source of antioxidants and nutrients. Bananas are the best!

Calendula

Calendula is a nourishing, moisturizing and wound-repairing herb. It's anti-inflammatory properties help reduce redness and provide relief from bug bites, scratches and other common skin irritations. The antiseptic, antibacterial and antiviral abilities of calendula make it a preferred natural remedy for skin irritations, wound healing, and even scar reduction. A calendula hair rinse will add shine and highlights to the hair while soothing the scalp.

Castor Oil

Castor oil is regarded by some as a natural remedy for soothing sore muscles as well as alleviating constipation. Folk healers around the world have long relied on this oil to treat a variety of ailments. This sticky substance is an effective emollient and overall healer, and is highly beneficial for health and wellness.

Chamomile

Chamomile is useful for almost all skin conditions and healing. Chamomile is also regarded for its powerful anti-inflammatory properties, and is useful for acne, rosacea, redness, bug bites, irritation, and more. A compress made from a cooled chamomile tea bag can reduce puffy and swollen eyes. The soothing tea or supplement promotes a sense of calm and relaxes you, so is ideal before bedtime.

Chia Seed

"Chia" is the Mayan word for strength, and it's no wonder! Apache and Aztec warriors sustained themselves by bringing these seeds on conquests for energy. More than just a clay figurine with sprouts for hair, Chia is rich in EFA's, protein, vitamins, soluble fiber and minerals, rendering it a superfood. Chia seeds can be ground into a powder for use in baking and cooking or added whole to smoothies, cereal and salads. They swell when added to water, making them super filling too!

Coconut Oil

Great for dry skin, cooking, smoothies and deep conditioning hair treatments, this oil is loaded with nourishing nutrients like lauric acid and triglycerides. It's great for cooking and adding to tons of yummy foods, as well as dry skin, and luscious locks. This tasty treat is great for overall health and wellness.

Cucumbers

The humble cucumber is filled with water, nutrients, vitamin C, and caffeic acid, which would explain why it has long been used as a topical treatment for swollen eyes and irritated skin. The anti-inflammatory and astringent properties can benefit a variety of skin ailments while hydrating, toning, and nourishing delicate tissue. Slices of this refreshing veggie can be applied directly to closed eyes to reduce puffiness in as little as 15 minutes. Just lie down and relax while the cool cucumber works its magic.

Cucumber may also be grated or liquefied and added to a base of witch hazel to create a soothing, astringent skin tonic. You should also add the wonder we know as cucumber to your salads, smoothies, soups, and more, as the high water content along with beneficial minerals are a must for glowing skin.

Frankincense (Olibanum)

Frankincense is renowned for sacred uses because it slows and deepens breath during meditation. The essential oil is also exceptional for mature skin due to its regenerative properties. Commonly used in traditional Indian medicine, Frankincense supplements are also indicated for joint pain, arthritis, colitis, asthma, sore throat, PMS, and even cancer.

Goji Berries

Goji berries are one of the richest sources of vitamins and other nutrients available. They contain over 18 different amino acids and vitamins such as B1, B2, B6, and E. This fruit is a natural source of vitamin C and contains more beta carotene (vitamin A) than carrots.

The dried berries are an awesome nutrient-filled snack or addition to your cereal. Pick this berry up in a powder form, to add to smoothies or your favorite recipes!

Gotu Kola (Centella asiatica)

This native plant from India has been used for centuries to treat inflammation, redness, burns and accelerate healing. Studies have shown that this amazing plant may also stimulate collagen synthesis and improve elasticity. It is also taken orally to treat a variety of ailments. Some also refer to Gotu Kola as Brahmi.

Grapeseed Oil

Grapeseed oil is a byproduct of wine making and loaded with wonderful antioxidants including powerful polyphenols, to combat free radical damage and protect the skin. This naturally occurring oil is great for all skin types including mature, oily, and even acne-prone skin. This dual-purpose oil is great topically, or as an ingredient in salad dressings and for cooking.

Hemp Seed Oil

This super sustainable oil is a highly nutritious food and contains antioxidants, protein, carotene, phytosterols and phospholipids, as well as a number of minerals. It is called a "complete protein" because it contains all nine essential amino acids. It is available in powder form for cooking and green beauty drinks. Topically, hemp seed oil has some of the highest content of essential fatty acids (EFAs) and linoleic acid, both of which not only provide nourishment to the skin but also aid in the healing and treatment of delicate skin conditions including eczema, acne, rosacea, and psoriasis.

Honey

The medicinal benefits of honey have long been recognized. Honey contains a multitude of vitamins and minerals and its antimicrobial properties help sooth sore throats and coughs. Also known for its antiseptic properties, honey can kill bacteria and help prevent infection. Honey can also relieve itchy, dry, irritated skin. Research supports the theory that the use of local raw honey can build an immunity to seasonal allergies. Honey added to chamomile tea may help to alleviate insomnia.

When you purchase honey, it should be from local, ethical beekeepers, because this kind of honey will contain the pollen from resident flowers and provide your body with what it needs to create antibodies to fight native allergens and bacteria. Honey can help boost your immune function, overall health, and resistance to infection.

Did you know that today honeybees are actually almost extinct? The use of chemicals and pesticides in traditional farming has lead to almost wiping out the entire bee population! So by purchasing local honey and organic foods, you are supporting not only your own health and beauty but also the sustainability of the environment.

Because honey is a natural humectant, it attracts moisture and helps retain balanced levels in the skin. It can be mixed with ground oats and aloe vera gel or avocado for a super soothing, hydrating mask. Its natural antibacterial properties are also useful for inflammation and acne. Just dab a bit directly on blemishes or reddened areas.

Kombucha

Kombucha is a drink made from sweetened tea that is fermented by a bacteria and yeast culture which results in a probiotic-filled drink. Probiotics are a "good" bacteria produced as a byproduct of the reaction between the tea and the other bacteria. Benefits of consuming these beneficial bacteria may include increased immunity, improved liver function and even the reduction of your risk of developing chronic illness like cancer. You can choose to make your own, but if you purchase Kombucha, choose a raw variety to ensure the cultures are present. Add some chia seeds to your drink and create an easy omega/probiotic drink!

Lavender Essential Oil

Lavender promotes the growth of new skin cells, making it highly regenerative. Lavender has a healing effect on burns, sunburn, acne, psoriasis, scarring, and even fungal growth. Excellent for red, irritated skin, lavender also alleviates stress and promotes restful sleep. Lavender will also repel pesky bed bugs and other irritating insects, so take a sachet with you when you travel!

Licorice Root

Licorice root has long been used in Ayurvedic medicine as a treatment for inflammation, burns, wounds and other general skin problems. It is very soothing to dry or irritated skin, reduces hyperpigmentation and discoloration and soothes skin. As a tea or supplement, it can help minimize adrenal stress and fatigue. But use with caution, if taken internally it can also raise blood pressure.

Lemon

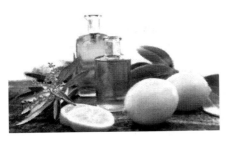

Lemons contain an abundance of vitamins and natural alpha-hydroxy acids that offer skin refining, brightening, and exfoliating properties. This wonder-fruit detoxifies the liver when added to warm water and offers benefits for everything from constipation to dental problems.

Lemons also offer higher levels of vitamin C than oranges and provide powerful antioxidant and antiseptic properties. Why not add organic lemon to your daily regimen? A lemon juice and water combination also makes a great all-natural house cleaning agent that smells heavenly!

Oats

Oatmeal baths are an ancient remedy for itchy skin, poison ivy, sunburn, rashes, dry skin and conditions such as psoriasis and eczema. Studies have shown the naturally-occurring constituents (good chemicals) in oatmeal have anti-inflammatory properties. Oatmeal softens and soothes the skin and is also a great source of fiber and antioxidants when added to your diet. Oats may help beat insomnia, improve metabolism, keep you regular, stabilize blood sugar, and lower cholesterol. Avoid "enriched" and "genetically modified" oats and consult a physician prior to use if you have Celiac disease or gluten sensitivity.

Olive Oil

Need a quick fix for dry, flaky skin? Grab the extra virgin olive oil! It imparts a healthy glow to your skin almost immediately. High quality extra virgin olive oil contains valuable vitamins and nutrients along with potent antioxidants that protect the body both internally and externally. The healthy fats in olive oil offer numerous health benefits.

Patchouli Essential Oil

An aromatic oil, patchouli stimulates collagen and elastin production reducing fine lines, wrinkles and even cellulite. Patchouli is also an anti-bacterial oil, which makes it a wonderful natural household cleanser. You can add a few drops to distilled water to disinfect your toilet, floors or just mist in the air with this wonderful, fragrant essential oil. But use caution, because this oil also acts as an aphrodisiac. So watch out! A few drops of patchouli will go a long way.

Peppermint Oil

Peppermint oil naturally alleviates headaches, migraines, and even nausea. Also indicated for hair loss, this miraculous plant repels insects and creates an uplifting, energizing experience if you are feeling sluggish. Tea, plant, or oils derived from peppermint are all wonderful. Just don't get the oil in your eyes, yowza!

Pomegranate

Pomegranate falls into the superfruit category because of its exceptional nutritional value and antioxidant properties. It contains age-defying ellagic acid, a powerful antioxidant, along with vitamin C. Recent research suggests that eating pomegranate may help reduce your risk of developing Alzheimer's disease and even cancer![26] Inside and out, this pure beauty offers benefits galore! The tea, juice, and powder forms make pomegranate super easy to incorporate into your daily regimen.

Rooibos Tea

Rooibos tea contains healthy amounts of iron, magnesium, zinc, and vitamin C, which are all essential for anti-aging and combating free radical damage. It also contains the antioxidant enzyme *superoxide dismutase,* which helps to ward off aging and cellular injury. You can create a beautiful body oil by infusing the loose tea into extra virgin olive oil. Simply strain the loose tea out after a few weeks and voila! You've got a super nourishing antioxidant-rich oil.

Rosemary

Rosemary has been used traditionally to stimulate hair growth and is often used to ease muscle pain. A powerful antioxidant, rosemary is able to neutralize harmful free radicals that damage skin cells for anti-aging effects. Rosemary also promotes circulation for a healthy-looking complexion and its fresh scent stimulates the nervous system. Rosemary is also great for household cleaning due to its antimicrobial properties.

Tea Tree Oil

Tea tree oil is a broad-spectrum anti-bacterial, anti-fungal and anti-viral agent used to treat a variety of infections. It is also highly effective for reducing blemishes, easing the sting of bug bites and killing toenail fungus. One of favorite my travel companions, tea tree is a super oil that treats just about anything.

Tomatoes

Tomatoes are a natural source of antioxidants, carotenoids, potassium, and lycopene. Orally, this superfood combats free radical damage and protects the skin from accelerated aging.

Topically, the citric acid content of tomatoes also offers natural exfoliating properties. Combine equal parts of fresh tomato juice and lemon juice and apply to blemishes for 15 minutes, then rinse thoroughly. For normal to dry skin, mash a ripe tomato with avocado and apply as a mask for 15 minutes, then rinse with warm water.

Turmeric

Turmeric is an amazing plant that adds incredible flavor to curry and other foods. The root of turmeric is also used widely for its medicinal properties. Turmeric is traditionally used orally for arthritis, stomach disorders, pain, headaches, and when applied to the skin, turmeric can help reduce inflammation, minimize bruising, and brighten the skin. Turmeric also has wonderful anti-cancer properties, and is gaining popularity as a chemopreventive and even a complementary chemotherapeutic.

Vitamin E

Vitamin E is a powerful antioxidant which helps to maintain youthful, healthy skin when applied topically. It also helps to promote healing and minimizes scars. Vitamin E that is sold in stores is not always natural, and instead is often synthetic. Opt for natural varieties when purchasing this super-nutrient and consider whole natural food sources such as almonds, sunflower seeds, turnips, peanut butter, argan oil, and safflower oil.

All-natural E in liquid form, such as d-alpha tocopherol is also available. Avoid a vitamin E product that has a "dl" prefix because that means it's a synthetic variety. Just a few drops of vitamin E in edible vegetable oils will help prevent them from going rancid quickly. That's pretty powerful stuff!

Witch Hazel

Witch hazel is widely used as an astringent to control sweat and oil production. It is also useful for treatment of bug bites, sores, blemishes, bruising, and swelling, and is even helpful for hemorrhoids and varicose veins. This super natural plant was traditionally used by American Indians for medicinal purposes and continues to be a staple in many household cabinets today. Double distilled organic witch hazel often has less alcohol, providing a more soothing version than most store-bought brands.

While there are many more naturally occurring topical and ingestible beauty aids, start incorporating these goodies into your regimen to experience some super beauty and wellness benefits!

Ayurveda – Ancient Natural Medicine for No Bull Beauty

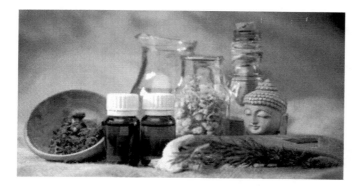

Taking it just another step further, natural remedies for healthy skin can extend beyond just a few plant-based skincare products and essential oils.

Ayurveda is an ancient Holistic Hindu system of medicine that incorporates mind and body exercises along with diet, topical and internal herbal treatments, and Yogic practice for healing and wellness. The term Ayurveda is a combination up of the words "Ayu" (meaning life) and "Veda" (meaning knowledge or science). Ayurveda is commonly referred to as "the science of life."

According to ancient Ayurvedic principles, there are three constitutional Doshas (unique mind and body types) – Vatta, Pitta, and Kapha. These are represented by elements from the Earth and are present in varying degrees within each person. According to Ayurvedic medicine, keeping the Doshas in balance is the key to health and wellness.

The Doshas and Their Relations to Your Skin Type

Vatta (Air and Ether) - Those with a primarily Vatta Dosha have skin that can be described as delicate, yet also dry and flaky. For those with this type, skin is often thin and although these individuals are more susceptible to signs of aging (like wrinkles and fine lines) they're also blessed with less acne and often that fine porcelain look coveted by many.

Vatta skin types are also usually prone to eczema and other skin irritations common to sensitive skin. These folks are drawn to warmth and light, so hydration is essential, as is consistent application of antioxidants, creams, and oils that soothe and protect this delicate skin type.

Pitta (Fire and Water) - Those with a dominant Pitta Dosha are quite opposite of those with Vatta. Pitta skin types crave coolness and their skin is easily aggravated by heat. As a result, those with Pitta skin are easily sunburned and have problems with inflammation, irritation, redness, etc.

Pitta skin is fair, often with freckles and/or moles, and is known to emit a warm glow. Pitta skin requires great care and is sensitive to the development of conditions such as rosacea, pigmentation, and rashes. This skin type should be supported with skincare products that help reduce inflammation, soothe, and prevent rosacea.

Kapha (Earth and Water) - Kapha skin is characterized by oiliness, large pores, and coolness to the touch. As a result, those with Kapha skin types are often prone to acne and blackheads but also have the benefit of thicker skin which helps delay the signs of aging, along with skin that feels very soft to the touch. These individuals often experience water retention, too, and must cleanse regularly to prevent breakouts and fungal infections.

Selecting Products for Your Ayurvedic Skin Type

Regardless of your Ayurvedic skin type, avoidance of synthetic products is essential, as they can create an imbalance. The Ayurvedic principles can be applied to your entire body system, and, when in balance, your skin will also go back in balance, as nature intended to achieve ultimate harmony. Examples of ancient Ayurvedic ingredients include gotu kola, neem, neroli, Bulgarian rose, sesame oil, jasmine, rosehip seed oil, sweet almond oil, frankincense, turmeric, sandalwood, and many more! Consultations with a professional experienced in both beauty and the art of Ayurveda can assist you in selecting the appropriate products for your Ayurvedic skin type.

Essential Oil Essentials

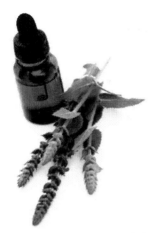

Many holistic practitioners have long revered essential oils for their capacity to relieve a variety of ailments. The therapeutic use of pure essential oils from plants is called aromatherapy. Numerous studies reveal the many health benefits of aromatherapy including a reduction of common symptoms of anxiety and depression as well as an improved quality of life for people facing chronic health conditions. Aromatherapy is now widely used in treatment centers to alleviate stress and worry, and even to help cancer patients feel calm and relaxed.

What Are Essential Oils?

Essential oils are the volatile oils derived from plant petals, leaves, stems, fruit rinds, and even barks. The pure, unadulterated oils contain active compounds that offer a multitude of benefits for healthy skin and hair, and also for a healthy mind. Therapeutic grade essential oils are antimicrobial, antifungal, antibacterial and also offer a multitude of other incredible benefits. Each individual oil offers its own unique properties and, when combined appropriately (by a specially trained aromatherapist) with complementing oils, offers a powerful synergy to treat a broad spectrum of ailments.

When applied to the skin, essential oils should be diluted and applied via a carrier oil or distilled water (and shaken well) to avoid skin sensitization or irritation. Carrier oils include olive oil, sesame seed oil, hemp seed oil, hazelnut, jojoba and avocado oil. Two common oils that can often be safely applied directly to the skin are lavender and tea tree oil. To avoid potential sensitivity it is recommended to dilute the lavender or tea tree oil in a carrier oil and patch test a small area of the skin. Properly diluted essential oils also offer non-toxic cleaning solutions for your home.

Another way to avoid potential irritation is to use hydrosol, a pure plant water that has similar properties to those of essential oils, but in a much less concentrated form. Hydrosols, also known as floral waters, distillates or hydrolats, are produced from the steam-distilling process of plants, and are typically a by-product of essential oil production.

Make certain that you purchase true, therapeutic grade essential oils. Many manufacturers adulterate essential oils by mixing them with synthetic oils to keep costs down. Another sneaky tactic! For optimum results only purchase high-quality, therapeutic grade oils that have not been processed, diluted, extracted with solvents or diluted with synthetic additives.

Hydrosols produced in small batches via organic methods offer the highest quality. When produced in this manner, they contain all of the essence of the plant, but in a diluted form making them more gentle and suitable for sensitive skin. Some examples of popular hydrosols used for soothing and rejuvenating the skin (and the mind) include Bulgarian rose damascena, chamomile, calendula, and neroli (orange blossom) hydrosols.

How Essential Oils Work

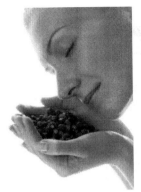 **So Here's the Deal:** Scent receptors send messages through your nervous system to the part of your brain that controls emotions. This makes essential oils useful for everything from stress relief to energizing. That being said, these oils are highly concentrated, and you do not want to get them in your eyes or apply them topically in their undiluted form.

Often aromatherapy is used in beauty products or during a massage to combine the healing properties of purification, moisturizing, cleansing, and relaxation. Don't be fooled by synthetic fragrance, which does not offer the same therapeutic properties. Only therapeutic grade essential oils safely offer aromatherapy benefits.

Aromatherapy provides many benefits, some of which include:

- Calming
- Stimulating
- Uplifting
- Anti-anxiety
- Emotional Healing
- PMS Reduction
- Stress Reduction

Some Popular Essential Oils for Aromatherapy

Common methods for aromatherapy include inhalation or diffusing essential oils. These oils are commonly used in aromatherapy, and are valued for the following therapeutic effects:

- **Bergamot** - Refreshing, uplifting. Reduces anxiety and stress.
- **Chamomile** - Calms nerves, promotes sleep and relaxation.
- **Clary Sage** - Calming, eases nerves and symptoms associated with menopause and PMS.
- **Frankincense** - Great for deepening the breath, meditation, and focus. A sacred oil.
- **Grapefruit** - Uplifting. Helps with stress and anxiety.
- **Lavender** - Promotes restful sleep. Eases emotions and nerves.
- **Lemon** - Uplifting, stimulating, and cleansing/detoxifying.
- **Sweet Orange** - Uplifting, calms anger and anxiety.
- **Peppermint** - Stimulating, refreshing. Reduces fatigue.
- **Rose Damascena** - Promotes calm, peace, and sleep. Helps with sadness, grieving, hormonal shifts and stress.
- **Rosemary** - Uplifting. Supports memory to overcome exhaustion.

Therapeutic and Topical Properties

I recommend the following oils for these common ailments. Keep in mind that when applying topically, these oils should first be diluted.

- **Hair Loss** - Rosemary, peppermint.
- **Toothache** - Clove, neem.
- **Fungus (feet and nails)** - Tea tree, eucalyptus, neem, rosemary.
- **Rashes** - German chamomile, lavender, rose, tea tree.
- **Muscle Aches** - Birch, wintergreen, marjoram, cypress, basil.
- **Headaches & Nausea** - Peppermint, rosemary, ginger, lavender.
- **Bug Repellant** - Tea tree, lavender, peppermint, lemongrass, eucalyptus.

Essential oils are good for just about everything from acne to household cleaning, so the list doesn't end here!

While there is so much more I can share about various essential oils and their properties, both alone and in combination, one of the most important things to remember is to always *use caution* when handling essential oils. They can easily irritate the eyes and skin if not diluted properly, and also stain clothing and furniture. You may even experience allergies to oils if you are sensitive to the plant from which they are derived. Essential oils can easily enter the body through inhalation and can cause sleepiness or be extremely stimulating. In addition, overuse may result in a paradoxical effect. Consult a professional for a personal consultation to be safe. Essential oils *are* essential in my opinion, as they offer so many benefits for you, your home, and much more!

Are You Loyal to Oil?

Contrary to popular belief, when you strip your skin of natural oils it sends a message to the oil glands to produce more oil to protect it. So, even your skin knows its protective barrier has been compromised and works hard to replenish it, creating a vicious cycle. This can result in acne for people with oily skin. For other skin types, a lack of natural oils can result in dryness and flakiness. Using natural oils on your skin helps to keep the skin supple and protected while preventing the natural reaction of your skin to produce more oil, often caused by soap and water.

So why fear oil? The introduction of mineral oil, a petroleum-based oil commonly used in beauty products as an inexpensive alternative to botanical oils, may be the culprit.

Mineral Oil

Used for years in cosmetics and skincare products, mineral oil is often added to cut costs, and consumers end up paying for this cost-cutting move in the form of side effects. In its original form, mineral oil is known as a pore-clogging culprit. It acts as a barrier and prevents the release of toxins, a normal and necessary function of the skin.

Physicians and beauticians who were aware of mineral oil's usage in personal care products commonly recommended "oil-free" products to avoid common side effects like allergies, skin irritation, and clogged pores. Mineral oil is also non-biodegradable and *not* environmentally friendly.

Having said that, harsh cleansers, soaps and astringents sold by big beauty brands strip the skin of natural and essential oils. Long-used ingredients, such as sulfates and surfactant gels make skin feel dry and tight. These harsh ingredients leave the skin unprotected, which can irritate and damage skin, as the main purpose of the skin's natural oil is to offer protection. Thus, it is necessary to replenish the skin's protective oils, but this should be approached in the right way.

Contrary to mineral oil, pure plant oils are rich in EFAs (essential fatty acids) and other nutrients. They continuously collect water and pull energy from the sun and atmosphere extracting amaaaazing micro-nutrients from the soil, which the plant magically transforms into therapeutic oils! Each and every botanical oil offers its own unique properties for every skin type. However, you must seek oils that are not refined, bleached, deodorized or otherwise stripped of their internal goodness.

Did you know that certain combinations of plant oils and essential oils have the ability to dissolve dirt, debris, and makeup from the skin and leave it hydrated and silky smooth? Many plant oils also kill bacteria and have regenerative properties. The skin absorbs oil perfectly and does not cause clogged pores or a greasy appearance when combined properly. Having always been an advocate of oil, I am thrilled with the recent surge in demand for oil-based products.

However, we must not forget that the skin also requires water-based ingredients and humectants to prevent trans-epidermal water loss. The No Bull Beauty Method recommends the use of oils for both your face and body, in conjunction with hydrating serums and/or creams and botanical toners. This balanced regimen helps prevent accelerated aging and renews skin.

Avoid high-foaming cleansers (surfactants) and choose products that are free of harsh, stripping chemical ingredients. Oils are loyal to us, and you can trust that the right oils will protect your overall health and your skin while also meeting dietary needs. So let's get back to nature, and be loyal to oil. You won't regret it!

Foods to Flush

Often when people experience a breakout or flaky skin, they quickly blame their skincare products, the environment or genetics. While these things may be partially responsible, it's important to also consider what you are consuming. Your diet has a profound effect on your appearance, and can determine whether your hair and skin condition is pretty or problematic. If you structure your diet around foods that are unprocessed and additive-free, then congratulations! You're on your way to having a lasting glow. If not, here are some foods you should avoid.

Saturated Fats

Meals with a high content of saturated fats have unfavorable consequences to your skin and health. Burgers, pizzas, and fried foods disrupt the health of your skin, making it highly reactive. These foods can cause inflammation, breakouts and even accelerate aging. It's not the food in its original form but the hydrogenated processed crap that's the culprit, and it's contributing to our environmental destruction too. Healthy fats and oils from plants, nuts, and seeds are great and healthy alternatives.

Processed Meats

Omit processed meats because they are loaded with salt and preservatives. The salt-additive duo will do nothing but seep moisture from your skin and also negatively impact your health. Even if store-bought sandwiches and convenience foods *seem* convenient, deli meats are believed to trigger skin inflammation. Do you really need to consume un-natural meat anyway? The hormones given to animals, such as androgens and IGF-1, have been shown to play a role in the development of adult and teenage acne by disrupting the natural hormone balance in people.[27]

In addition, they are responsible for greenhouse gases and compromise our planet. Glowing skin can be achieved by replacing (any or all) meat with healthy fats from unmodified sources that offer beauty benefits like nothing else!

Sweets Are Not so Sweet

No matter how sweet tasting these goodies are, highly processed sugary foods can break down the skin's collagen and elastin – two significant fibers that are responsible for making the skin plump and youthful. If these fibers deteriorate drastically, expect premature wrinkles and other age-related challenges.

It is important to realize that sweets can also contribute to other serious health issues. Processed sugars, white flour and starches including white potatoes are foods to flush, as they convert to sugar in the body and wreak havoc on your cells. In addition, many sugary foods contain gluten, which is a common problem today for millions of people and pets.

If you are not gluten sensitive, I'd suggest switching to 100 percent whole grains. Everyone should avoid foods that say "enriched" (which means stripped of nutrients) as well as "hydrogenated."

Curb the Caffeine and Alcohol

Alcoholic beverages may result in dryness and vasodilatation wherein the skin's blood vessels swell. This may result in broken capillaries. Alcohol also exacerbates inflammatory skin conditions such as rosacea.

I'm sorry to report that your daily espresso and frappuccino may also be leaching your skin's moisture. If you want to hydrate properly, choose water (and *not* in plastic bottles), or opt for antioxidant-rich teas and add a squeeze of lemon to detoxify. A healthy drink will make a world of difference for your skin and body.

Ditch the Dairy

Dairy has long been accused of contributing to clogged pores and whiteheads (milia). High-fat dairy products can also increase acne as well as promote inflammation. Dairy products surely cloud an otherwise clear complexion and contribute to phlegm and mucus. This is because dairy products (particularly full fat varieties) may actually prompt the body to produce more androgens. Androgens are hormones that can cause your body to produce extra oil and sebum, which clogs pores. Not something anyone wants, especially if his or her skin is already prone to acne.

Veggies like spinach and other leafy greens supply the calcium you need without these unwanted side effects. You can also select almond, flax, or rice milk and obtain all the wonderful nutrients from these more advantageous drinks for healthier skin.

Goodbye to Gluten

Gluten is a grain found in wheat, oats, barley, and rye. So why do does this natural food pose such a problem? It may not, in your case, but gluten is often a culprit of many disorders that you may have overlooked. If you suffer from bowel problems, chronic pain, recurring sinus issues, irritability, resistant skin conditions, or any pesky annoyances, consider omitting gluten from your diet for a few weeks to see how you feel.

Gluten-free is a growing trend for good reason. Celiac disease is a serious auto-immune disease in which the grain invaders cause an immune reaction that attacks the small intestines, leading to discomfort, nutrient deficiencies, and even cancer. Fortunately, "gluten-free" foods are available in abundance today, and while not always as tasty, they may just change your life.

Other 'Bad Boys' to Avoid

- Artificial flavors
- Artificial sweeteners (Splenda®, aspartame, ace-k, neotame, saccharin, etc.)
- Artificial colors
- High-fructose corn syrup
- MSG (monosodium glutamate, flavor enhancer, hydrolyzed protein)
- Trans Fats (labeled as shortening, partially hydrogenated or hydrogenated oils)
- Preservatives (BHT/BHA, TBHQ, sulfites, polysorbate, etc.)

Many of these ingredients can lead to a host of health problems, including heart disease, diabetes, high cholesterol, auto-immune disease, and some cancers. Do your best to eliminate hydrogenated fats, refined sugars, white flour, and all processed foods. These highly processed foods can elevate blood sugar, leading to skin inflammation, which also accelerates aging. Try parting ways with the above-mentioned foods and see the changes for your skin, scalp, and overall health.

Viva La Veggies

The vegan diet trend is quickly sweeping the nation for a variety of reasons such as the many health benefits, beauty advantages, cruelty-free compassion and environmental concerns.

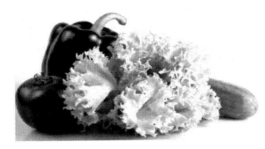

If you have not observed the various celebrities, politicians, and many others following this diet, you should Google it! Natalie Portman, Ellen DeGeneres, Alyssa Milano, Brad Pitt, Prince, and former President Bill Clinton are just a few celebrities who opt for the vegan lifestyle. There are numerous reasons they are making the change.

Here are just a few good reasons to try a vegan diet, which is endorsed by many famous folks and health experts:

Beauty Benefits

Did you ever think that omitting dairy and meat from your diet could support your natural beauty? Many sources say it can! The hormones in meat can change your own hormone balance and contribute to many skin and health challenges.

As mentioned previously, dairy can also cause clogged pores and create more mucus, which causes inflammation of the skin and additional challenges. Substitute with water and veggies when you can. It is important to maintain a healthy, balanced diet. If you are considering transitioning to a plant-based diet, you should seek the advice of a nutritionist.

Positive Global Effect

More than healthy food, having a vegan diet greatly contributes to a sustainable environment. Experts say that meat and dairy products call for more preparation, involve hormonal and antibiotic drug use, and result in the highest greenhouse-gas emissions on our planet. Meat-based foods all have magnified carbon footprints in comparison to plant-based foods. Rather than bingeing on fatty and high cholesterol foods, you can opt for climate-friendly foods that also contribute to saving the planet.

Lower Risk for Disease

Physicians and nutritionists agree that a plant-based diet is optimal for good, lasting health.[28] Cattle and dairy farms often inject their livestock with hormones and antibiotics, which contribute to numerous challenges when ingested by humans. There is no doubt that what we are doing is not natural. Problematic blood pressure, heart diseases, and particular forms of cancer have all been associated with large intakes of meat when compared to vegetable-based diets, in combination with genetic factors and sedentary lifestyles.

If you decide to go veggie, remember to transition slowly and seek professional guidance to ensure you do not send your system into shock.

Cruelty-Free Compassion and Environmental Impact

Minimizing your environmental impact through a vegan (or vegetarian) diet is a great thing. Moreover, while modern living allows animal testing, genetic modification, and other cruel practices, these diets can offer you a sense of quiet satisfaction. It just feels good to know that you are actively making changes that support the health of other living creatures, and the environment. You'll be improving your health and promoting your own natural beauty from the inside out.

Most people don't know what animals endure as a result of modern living and personal lifestyle choices, and it can be hard to swallow. The environmental impact of the mass production of meats, like clear-cutting of rainforest land to provide grazing pastures for cattle, the amount of oil that it takes to transport the meat, and hormones/chemicals in the meats needed to create the amount of food that is in demand, all have dramatic negative effects on our environment. They also negatively affect your whole body, from your skin to digestion, immune health, and overall wellness.

Widened Palate

Contrary to common belief, vegans enjoy a lot of yummy dishes! With hundreds of veggies and non-dairy alternatives available at local markets today, you will never run out of exciting foods to try.

The abundance of omega fatty acids, vitamins, and nutrients from green foods and fruits not only benefit us internally, but externally too when we radiate from clearer skin, more even-toned skin and a feeling of happiness. From salads to main dishes, you will find lots of resources for cool new recipes, and you don't have to feel guilty when you overeat!

While a vegan lifestyle may not be your preference, I am simply sharing the benefits of a plant-based diet, as so many of my clients ask me why this trend is so popular. If you desire to transition to a vegetarian or vegan diet, consult with a qualified nutritionist or your healthcare provider to ensure your nutrient and vitamin B12 levels are sufficient.

As a professional, I am often asked for my recommendations on beauty, and the truth is that often times omitting dairy and meat can make a world of difference. At a minimum, I do recommend you omit the hormone and antibiotic treated meats, fish, and dairy from your diet and replace them with organic, free-range, hormone and drug-free meat options. Not only will you look and feel better, but you'll be doing our planet a favor.

Cuckoo for Coconuts?

Have you wondered why so many people are in a coconut craze? With the abundance of chemically treated foods and confusing choices, you may be limited; however, you can never go wrong with coconuts.

Coconuts offer numerous benefits at an affordable price. Coconuts are filled with lauric acid, which is considered a potent antibacterial and antiviral agent. In fact, Ayurvedic medicine relies on coconut for its power in warding off harmful bacteria. Coconut can also naturally help strengthen your immune system.

Coconut water is a great option for hydration, particularly after strenuous workouts, as it offers nutrients that water alone does not supply. And it tastes yummy! Make sure to consider the caloric intake though if weight loss or maintenance is a desire for you.

Coconut oil assists in moisturizing the skin, and when combined with other effective ingredients, you can achieve the perfect synergy. When it comes to skin care, coconut oil offers benefits both inside and out, as it contains unique fatty acids called triglycerides that nurture skin both topically and orally. Only raw organic virgin coconut oil supplies the nutrients and benefits needed for super skin and hair, so be sure to read your labels.

Coconut oil has long been used as a hair conditioner, but it's also an all-in-one product that makes the hair stronger, silkier, and shinier while keeping it free from dandruff. Massaging the scalp with coconut oil can provide benefits for healthier hair production but, it can weigh down thin, fine hair so make sure to start with a tiny amount. You can always add more.

You can use organic virgin coconut oil topically or incorporate it in your diet, for all of the great health benefits it has to offer. Adding this superfood to any No Bull Beauty Smoothie or simply ingesting one or two tablespoons of organic virgin coconut oil a day can also promote healthy skin and hair from the inside out. The anti-inflammatory properties of coconut make it a super beauty supplement.

While the Philippines is the world's largest exporter of virgin coconut oil, it's a relief to know that products manufactured from this fruit are not difficult to find wherever you are. However, it cannot be obtained in pill form as easily.

Super Duper Beauty Boosters

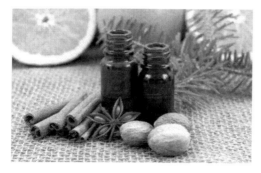 As we have discussed, one of the secrets to beautiful skin and hair is proper nutrition. The foods you eat can and will eventually show on the outside. Why is this?

Your internal organs such as your liver, kidneys, adrenals, thyroid, and intestines are responsible for breaking down the food you consume and for eliminating toxins. If your diet is less than ideal, you are putting pressure on these organs. And remember, your skin is the largest elimination organ of the body so an unhealthy diet and poor quality products can lead to breakouts, dry skin, and accelerated aging. Here are some easy-to-use foods that can help you to achieve more beautiful, radiant, and healthy skin.

Easy Peasy Lemon Squeezy!

Lemons, and other citrus fruits like oranges and grapefruits contain unique antioxidant compounds including limonoids and flavonoids that offer powerful protection against pre-mature aging. These compounds have been shown to aid in the prevention of all kinds of cancer and other chronic illnesses. Lemons are especially rich in vitamin C along with other nutrients that detoxify the liver, enhance the immune system and stimulate vital organs to function optimally, including the skin.

Vitamin C is one of the healthiest nutrients you can provide your skin. This vitamin aids in the production of collagen, an essential structural component of healthy, youthful skin. Reduced collagen content can lead to sagging, fine lines, wrinkles, and much more. Vitamin C also helps fight free radical damage due to its potent antioxidant properties. So, start your day with a fresh squeezed organic lemon in a glass of warm water to purify your skin and body, and promote a healthy glow!

Of course, you can also obtain vitamin C from a multitude of other foods. These include fruits and veggies like, oranges, grapefruit, limes, blueberries, goji berries, pomegranate, acai berry, strawberries, red bell peppers, broccoli and brussels sprouts. In general, the brighter or richer the color, the higher the antioxidant content.

Get Your Greens On

Leafy green veggies are not just a way to incorporate vegetables into your diet, they're also an easy way to improve health and radiate beauty. Leafy green vegetables contain micro-nutrients only found in plants, along with fiber, vitamins and minerals. Some of the top greens for health and wellness include: kale, collards, turnip greens, swiss chard, spinach, seaweed, broccoli and red and green leaf romaine lettuce. Whether you add them to your smoothies or incorporate them into daily meals or salads, your skin, hair and body will appreciate it.

Herbs and Spice… Oh-So Nice!

Inside and out, herbal remedies and commonly used spices can provide a variety of beauty benefits. For example, adding herbs and spices like cumin, garlic, turmeric, sage, rosemary, and thyme, to your meals not only enhances flavor but also provides you with minerals and nutrients galore to enhance and support the immune system, and the health of your entire body, including your skin.

Teas or tinctures of holy basil, lotus, cinnamon, red clover, lemon balm, catnip, reishi mushroom, peppermint, burdock, and ginger, amongst many other organically grown herbs offer a multitude of health benefits to combat the formation free-radicals, alleviate pain, reduce stress, fight disease and prevent accelerated aging.

Some of the more popular teas including rooibos, pomegranate, acai, white and green tea also support health and wellness naturally through their powerful antioxidants including polyphenols, catechins and flavonoids that improve the immune system's functions and the body as a whole. Like many of the herbs mentioned previously, these teas also protect the skin from free radicals that often lead to chronic health issues and premature aging.

Prepare your beauTEAS as you would any other cup of tea. Add fresh herbs to hot water, seep for about 10-15 minutes covered, strain and enjoy! You can also cool tea and enjoy these wonderful herbs over ice. If you desire a touch of sweetness, avoid sugar and choose a natural sweetener like raw honey or Stevia (unprocessed), and add a squeeze of lemon for the perfect synergy.

Nutritious Nuts and Super Seeds

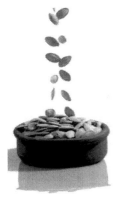

Many nuts and seeds are rich in omega fatty acids, protein, and other essential nutrients for healthy skin including zinc. Almonds, walnuts, flax, chia, and sunflower seeds are great protein and omega fatty acid sources for everyone, including vegans and vegetarians. Pumpkin seeds and peanuts are great sources of both omega fatty acids and zinc.

Zinc helps to metabolize testosterone, a component responsible for producing sebum, the overproduction of which contributes to acne. Omega fatty acids help the skin by fighting common problems like dryness and inflammation. Try snacking on healthy nuts and seeds to see a difference in your skin, hair and health.

Water-Based Foods

Water is an essential nutrient, especially for your skin. Since water is in every cell, and your skin is made up of over 50 percent water, getting the recommended amount of this nutrient is very important when it comes to the health and beauty of your skin. But you don't have to choke down 8 tall glasses a day just to get the water your body needs! Water-dense fruits and vegetables can also increase your water intake. Try snacking on cucumbers, broccoli, celery, melon or tomatoes. Natural whole foods have the highest water content. They also provide fiber and other nutrients that keep skin supple, youthful, and radiant! In addition to drinking your water, you can also start "eating your water."

All of these beauty-boosting foods are wonderful alone, but a simple way to incorporate all the fresh foods you need is through this incredibly tasty and healthy No Bull Beauty Smoothie. This simple drink is packed full of nature's goodness, to restore your youthful radiance and protect against free radical damage. Try it for yourself and switch it up with any substitutions or changes you prefer. Experience just how tasty natural beauty can be!

No Bull Beauty Smoothie

Ready for a diet makeover that works from the inside out for natural beauty? Add this delicious smoothie to your daily intake of healthy foods, including lots of fresh fruits and vegetables, and you'll be well on your way to supple skin, shiny hair, and radiant beauty - *No Bull*!

Ingredients:

- **Organic Blueberries** - Excellent source of antioxidants.
- **Organic Acai Berry** - A superfood, high in vitamin C content and omega fatty acids.
- **Organic Banana** - Add for potassium, super nutrients, texture and flavor!
- **Organic Chia Seeds** - A rich source of omega fatty acids & fiber to fight free radicals, fill you up and help you "go!"
- **Organic Hemp Powder** - A good source of protein and nutrients. Called a "complete protein" because it contains all 9 non-essential amino acids.

- **Organic Spirulina Powder** - Rich in vitamins, minerals, protein and amino acids for skin cell regeneration and health.
- **Organic Pomegranate Powder** - High in vitamin C and flavonoid antioxidants for super skin and health.
- **Organic Coconut Water or Water** - Coconut water contains electrolytes that are highly beneficial, but water of course has no flavor and no calories.
- **Organic Kale** - This leafy-green veggie provides large doses of a variety of different vitamins and minerals including iron.
- **Organic Rosehips** - High in vitamins A and C, to combat free radical damage.

Any way you shake it, this No Bull Beauty Smoothie will fill you with vitamins and essential nutrients that help your skin and hair look amazing from the inside out!

If you are new to juicing, blending, and creating smoothies, follow this basic recipe:

- **Blueberries** - 1/2 cup
- **Acai Berry Powder, or Juice** - 1 scoop or ½ cup
- **Banana** - 1 large banana, ripened
- **Chia Seeds** - 1/3 cup
- **Hemp Powder** - 1 scoop
- **Pomegranate Powder** - 1 scoop
- **Coconut Water** - 1 cup
- **Kale** - 1-2 heaping handfuls, rinsed
- **Rosehips** - Dried ground powder 1 Tbsp, or 1 heaping handful, fresh

- **Spirulina** - 1 Tbsp
- **Water to thin**

Directions:

1. Toss in all raw fruit, including blueberries and banana.
2. Mix chia seeds with 1 cup filtered water. Wait a few minutes, stir, and toss in blender.
3. Pulse blender. Add all powders, including hemp powder, acai, spirulina, and pomegranate powder.
4. Pulse blender. Add coconut water, and pulse again.
5. Add kale, rosehips, and water to thin.

Voila! Try this recipe if you're new to making smoothies, and from there, you can add any of the healthy-skin ingredients mentioned earlier. Everyone is different, so if you prefer different varieties and amounts, go for it!

Beauty Supplements and Superfood Sources

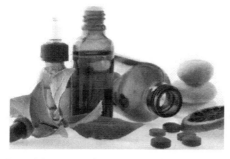

It is always my suggestion and utmost preference to obtain important nutrients via a healthy diet that includes fresh No Bull Beauty Smoothies, and whole, natural food sources but it's not always possible. So if you can't, try to get these superfoods as supplements from high-quality manufacturers that do not use fillers, binders, dyes, or chemicals in their formulas.

Ashwagandha

Many wonderful supplements such as tinctures, homemade tonics, and Ayurvedic herbs support the adrenal glands to reduce stress and increase your vitality! If stress is a problem for you, remember that it ages you, so consider adding Ayurvedic supplements or pure herbs of ashwagandha or brahmi to your daily regimen.

Astaxanthin

Astaxanthin is a potent anti-inflammatory agent and free-radical scavenger, rendering it a powerful anti-aging supplement. It belongs to the carotenoid family, which offer the bright color to foods such as beets, peppers, and salmon. However, astaxanthin is considered the most powerful source of carotenoids. This, along with unique antioxidant properties, enables astaxanthin to filter into every cell and provide numerous benefits for overall health and beauty.

Recent studies suggest that supplementing with astaxanthin may protect the skin by improving skin moisture levels and providing smoothness while minimizing fine lines and wrinkles. The anti-inflammatory properties assist in alleviating joint pain and UV damage.

This particular supplement must be harvested properly to ensure the highest quality, so choose a reputable manufacturer and select natural, non-animal microalgae-derived varieties.

Vitamin B Complex

Deficiencies in B vitamins can result in dry and dull skin, acne, wrinkles, rashes, splitting nails, and hair loss. Many women are deficient in B vitamins, so supplementation is helpful. The B-vitamin biotin in particular plays a role in hair health; 500 mcg (5mg) daily can make a big difference for thinning and sparse hair. Vitamin B6 converts EFAs into prostaglandins, an active chemical within the body that assists in controlling inflammation, which we want to be sure to keep at bay. Natural sources of B vitamins include spinach, potatoes, asparagus, peas, carrots and broccoli.

Vitamin C

Vitamin C is known as the "master antioxidant." This super vitamin protects and repairs skin cells. It doesn't only boost your immune system, but it helps to combat those pesky free radicals that attack healthy cells and contribute to pre-mature aging. Vitamin C promotes healthy skin, bones, eyes, and blood vessels.

If you opt for a supplement, choose one with bioflavonoids. Bioflavonoid antioxidants are often present in the same food sources as vitamin C. These flavonoids are what give fruits and vegetables their vibrant color. This "dynamic duo" of vitamin C and bioflavonoids are an antioxidant powerhouse that should be a part of your diet. Natural, fresh sources of vitamin C are lemons, pomegranates, acai berries, goji berries, tomatoes, and green and leafy vegetables.

Cacao (Raw Chocolate)

Raw Cacao, or unprocessed chocolate, is one of nature's best sources of pure plant polyphenols, fiber, and antioxidants. These compounds combat free radical damage and support a healthy circulatory system and overall cardiovascular function. Recent studies also suggest that the digestive enzymes may also help control blood pressure, cholesterol, and blood glucose levels.

Cacao fiber may keep you regular, which is essential for the removal of toxins from the system. A healthy circulatory system is essential for vibrant skin and hair. As little as 6.6 grams of cacao fiber sprinkled on your cereal, added to coconut water or milk (yum), or snacked on may be enough to do the trick! Finally, an excuse to have chocolate!

Coenzyme Q10

Coenzyme Q10 (CoQ10) plays a vital role in the production of collagen and other proteins for youthful looking skin. CoQ10 can help maintain overall skin elasticity and integrity, and dramatically reduce the signs of aging. By functioning as a powerful antioxidant and free radical scavenger, CoQ10 can also enhance your skin's natural defense system against environmental stress. CoQ10 is present in peanut butter, soybeans, and soybean oil. It also promotes heart health.

Ginger Root

Ginger is a powerful anti-inflammatory indicated for many annoying ailments. Known to alleviate nausea, bellyaches, and irritable bowel syndrome, this super root is readily available and a must for all household cabinets. Ginger has also been indicated for arthritis, fevers, nausea, toothaches, coughs, bronchitis, pain relief, and headaches. It helps to lower cholesterol, regulate blood pressure, and more! Ginger's anti-inflammatory abilities make it a great choice for beauty topically and internally, as well as anti-aging, as it softens skin and fights wrinkles due to its high vitamin C content.

Green Tea

Since free radicals cause skin damage which can result in signs of aging like fine lines, wrinkles, discoloration, and loss of elasticity, the high amounts of antioxidants in green tea supplements can help minimize the damage. The unique compound in green tea (EGCG) may also help with rosacea, and even acne. Try the tincture or fresh brewed tea to obtain maximum benefits.

Kelp and Seaweed

Packed with vitamins, trace minerals and antioxidants, these leafy sea vegetables also contain micro-nutrients like chlorophyll, essential fatty acids (EFAs), and proteins to help detoxify the body and improve your skin's ability to heal. Kelp, in supplement form supports the healthy function of your thyroid gland (a gland responsible for the production of hormones to promote cellular metabolism) and is a good source of iodine. As a beauty supplement, kelp restores moisture levels, firms the skin, nourishes, balances and hydrates. Kelp is also beneficial for luxurious hair.

You can also try kelp noodles, seaweed salads, or nori strips to obtain these vital nutrients. However, be advised that allergies to these types of foods are some of the most common, so check with your doctor before adding these sea veggies to your diet.

Magnesium

This super supplement is essential for bones, skin, regularity, anxiety, PMS, and the absorption of vitamin D, calcium, and more! Magnesium promotes optimal moisture levels in the skin and promotes healthy elasticity. It makes teeth and bones harder and stronger. A deficiency of magnesium can lead to a whole host of health and skin issues and also contribute to body odor. Supplementation is most beneficial in powder or liquid form so that you can vary your dose and work up slowly. Food sources of magnesium include sea vegetables, kelp, peanuts, almonds and brown rice.

Melatonin

Melatonin is a powerful antioxidant produced within the body. Unfortunately, levels of naturally-produced melatonin decline with age, leaving adults with limited antioxidant protection. Supplementing with melatonin not only assists with a better night's sleep, but recent research also suggests adding this supplement may help protect against common diseases including Alzheimer's, Parkinson's, and even stroke!

Melatonin may also provide relief from headaches and pain. Just be aware that melatonin does not work like a sleeping pill, and you'll need to take these supplements regularly as melatonin works to regulate your sleep pattern, not just put you to sleep.

MSM

A naturally occurring nutrient found in plants, meats, dairy products, fruits, and vegetables such as broccoli, peppers, cabbage, and other cruciferous veggies, MSM (methylsulfonylmethane) is nature's beauty fluid. It provides both aging skin and body with the building blocks needed to re-build strong and healthy collagen and elastin. MSM has been said to decrease the appearance of wrinkles, pigmentation (brown spots) and spider veins. Additional sources are sunflower seeds, soybeans, and garlic.

Omega Fatty Acids and GLA

Omega fatty acids are crucial for many body processes and offer numerous health and beauty benefits. These essential fatty acids (EFAs) are "essential" because the body does not produce them; they must be obtained through diet or supplementation. EFAs include omega 3, 6, 9, and omega-7. GLA (gamma-linolenic acid) is an omega-6 fatty acid particularly beneficial for anti-aging due to its anti-inflammatory properties. GLA has been effective in treating some of the most sensitive of skin conditions. Oils with high levels of GLA include evening primrose, hemp seed, and borage oils, which combat hair loss, dry skin, and symptoms of menopause. A super whole food source of GLA is spirulina (microalgae). When taking EFAs in supplement form, choose a high-quality supplement that undergoes quality assurance testing. And of course, remember to maintain a proper balance of omega-3 and omega-6 fatty acids.

Probiotics

Probiotics are live microorganisms that support the body's overall immune function via the digestive system. They work by ensuring that the body absorbs only the important food and nutrients during the digestive process. Furthermore, they support the breakdown and elimination of toxins and carcinogens in the body. A high-quality probiotic can make a world of difference.

Resveratrol and Grapeseed Extract

Resveratrol and grapeseed extract are anti-inflammatory agents and high-powered antioxidants derived from grapes. For this reason, they are known for their protective powers against harsh chemicals and free radicals that contribute to aging and disease. A well-known source of resveratrol is red wine, but keep in mind that red grapes by themselves are a better source. As we cannot easily consume the amount of wine or grapes needed to achieve desirable levels, organic resveratrol (or grapeseed extract supplements) will offer you the potency needed for age-defying benefits. Research suggests resveratrol offers a more concentrated form of grapeseed extract. The unique kind of antioxidant contained in grapes is called a polyphenol, and is one of the most powerful out there.

Also contained in blueberries, blackberries, and cranberries, this compound is found in the skin, and seeds of grapes.

Saw Palmetto, Evening Primrose, Milk Thistle, Chasteberry, and Black Cohosh

These herbs offer a natural alternative to hormone replacement. Natural herbal remedies are a great way to get through male or female-specific problems. Try them out to support a healthy libido, to ease PMS symptoms or ease menopause imbalances caused by hormones. There are a variety of herbal blends, so seek professional advice to determine which herbal supplement(s) may be best suited for your particular age and symptoms.

Spirulina

Spirulina is one of the most nutrient-rich superfoods on Earth. A member of the sea vegetable family, this blue-green microalgae is a natural source of protein, amino acids and iron along with a potent blend of vitamins A, C, B12, and many minerals.

This natural anti-inflammatory, immunity booster, and free radical inhibitor has also been shown to play a role in lowering the risk for age-related diseases. Due to spirulina's ability to increase cellular metabolism, it supports healing, and faster regeneration of skin cells. Since it's also packed with nutrients that support detoxification of the body, spirulina also helps reduce acne breakouts.

Triphala

Triphala is a combination of the potent Ayurvedic healing herbs: amalaki, bibhitaki, and haritaki. Considered the most effective colon tonic by alternative medicine practitioners, this herbal supplement blend of super fruits rejuvenates the skin and body via deep cleansing and purification. Triphala also increases resistance to daily stressors. It is best to consult with your physician prior to considering a cleansing herbal supplement.

Zinc

Zinc is an essential mineral that plays an important role in your body's cellular metabolism, immune function, growth, and wound healing. Acne sufferers often have a zinc deficiency, and a simple zinc supplement may significantly improve their skin condition.[29] However, too much zinc can create a copper imbalance, so have your levels checked regularly. Zinc occurs naturally in peanuts, kidney beans, dark chocolate, and pumpkin seeds.

When you consume vitamins from natural sources they're more readily available and easily used by your skin, and therefore are much more beneficial than their chemically derived counterparts. Always check with your physician prior to using them, please!

And of course Vitamin D....

To D or Not to D

Vitamin D is an essential component of a healthy body. Low levels of vitamin D have been linked to several health issues like heart disease, cancer, autoimmune disease, and even depression. Recent studies suggest that low vitamin D levels may contribute to rosacea, hair loss, and even heavy wrinkling. Vitamin D is also a hormone and is involved in the regulation of everything in the body. Because hormone imbalances contribute to a variety of skin conditions, it makes sense that a vitamin D deficiency would wreak havoc.[30] As we age, our bodies produce less vitamin D, so it is important to address this in order to protect and preserve your health and beauty. Since not everyone gets an ample supply of this delightful D vitamin, supplements are being recommended left and right.

The unfortunate news is that not all supplements are the same; some of them can be confusing. The question is, will you opt for D or not?

When selecting your D supplements, you need be informed that there are two options: vitamin D2 (ergocalciferol) and vitamin D3 (cholecalciferol). Vitamin D3 is commonly sourced from animals and is not vegetarian or vegan, but new plant-based options have recently been introduced. Vitamin D2 is synthetic (and vegan), but is only 69 percent as bio-available as vitamin D3. Therefore, your daily requirement may be greater if you select D2. This is important to know when selecting your supplement. You may also select a liquid or sub-lingual version for enhanced potency.

When it all comes down to it, the most appropriate (yet controversial) way for the body to have adequate levels of vitamin D is through sun exposure. Just 15 minutes daily is often enough, depending on your geographical location. The natural oils produced by your skin offer some protection, so it is best not to wash the skin right before a short exposure. Contrary to the common belief, a bit of sun exposure is not always to blame for skin cancer. Sunburns are actually the bigger culprits. Prolonged exposure can lead to burns, which is why balance is the key if you're after vitamin D. Be sure to wear toxin-free SPFs for any prolonged time outdoors. This way, you need not suffer the consequences of overexposure.

You may also indulge in vitamin D-enriched foods. Few foods naturally contain vitamin D. Fortified cereals, soymilk, and even fortified orange juice provide most of the vitamin D in American diets. Plant sources include sunflower seeds, alfalfa, sarsaparilla, and spinach. Additional foods rich in vitamin D include salmon, and milk, although hormone-treated cattle and farm-raised fish certainly have their contraindications for both health and beauty. Mushrooms are a great source of vitamin D. In some mushrooms, vitamin D is being boosted by exposing them to UV light, making them a viable option for those following a vegan or vegetarian diet. Some yeasts offer vitamin D, but often not in sufficient quantities to meet daily requirements. The body has to have vitamin D to make vitamin D. There is not a reserve, and therefore it must continuously be replenished.

The right dosage of vitamin D varies for each person. Several factors, including a person's weight and blood serum levels, must be examined to determine how much vitamin D is needed. The best way to find out your recommended intake is to have your levels tested. Many physicians order the wrong test, and when results come back showing sufficient levels, you may be overlooking something serious. The 25-hydroxy vitamin D blood test is the most accurate way to measure how much vitamin D is in your body.

Low levels of vitamin D can contribute to a weak immune system, later leading to other health challenges or diseases, so it's better to be safe than sorry. It is also thought that low levels contribute to the autoimmune skin condition psoriasis, which is partially why the treatment for that condition is light therapy. Ah-ha!

Taking vitamin D supplements is something you should first seek medical advice for. While some reports suggest that high doses can be harmful, recent research shows that those doses are extremely high and very unlikely. Vitamin D is also curiously forgiving in that you can make up for a missed dose by doubling up or even taking a week's worth at once. Make sure that you seek the guidance of experts so you can decide whether to D or not to D!

Other Benefits of Vitamin D

Vitamin D helps prevent osteoporosis, symptoms of depression, and some cancers, especially breast cancer. Studies show that a deficiency of this vitamin may contribute to diabetes, Alzheimer's, schizophrenia, and obesity.[31] Vitamin D deficiency can also result in hair loss and certain skin conditions. Keep in mind that wearing sunscreen blocks your body's ability to absorb and utilize vitamin

D from sunlight. So, if you're wearing sunscreen or sunblock every day, you may need a daily vitamin D supplement.

For some people, skin and hair issues result from thyroid, vitamin D or magnesium deficiencies. Please seek medical attention for proper blood work and analysis in these cases.

Somethin' Fishy 'Bout Fish Oil

Omega fatty acids are considered essential fatty acids and are great for skin, hair, heart and overall health. Everyone loves beauty and health supplements but the problem is, some folks are eating or taking higher levels of omega-6 fatty acids then omega-3. It is essential to have a healthy balance of both omega-6 and omega-3s. Your body does not produce these fatty acids (why they're called essential), so you need to obtain them from food sources. Omega-6 fats boost cell growth, blood clotting, and your body's natural immune response to inflammation. On the other hand, omega-3 fats control cell growth, decrease blood clotting, and minimize inflammation. It's easy to see why we need a balance of both.

Omega-6 comes from many plant oils, including acai berry, avocados, seaweed, and more. Omega-3 sources include chia seeds, flax seeds and walnuts. They are also abundant in oily fish and algae. Instead of eating these superfoods however, many people are taking omega-3 supplements via liquids, gels and capsules. A diet rich in balanced EFAs helps keep your skin smooth and supple, but is popping a fish oil capsule an easy way to make this happen? 'Cause there's something fishy about these supplements.

Because they are derived from fish, carnivores, vegetarians and vegans alike have reason for concern. Over-fishing is a problem for our fragile ecosystem, as is the contamination of our water from farm-raised fish. If your supplements are derived from farm-raised fish, the health benefits are diminished. As a result of the poor grain diet they are often fed, they lack the vital nutrients from algae and seaweed, and simply don't get the nutrients they need to supply you with those essential fats in the highest quality. Another challenge is heartburn. Nobody likes a fishy burp. Why does this happen anyway? Unfortunately, many fish oil capsules are rancid because fish oil is unstable.

Alternatively, consider oils such as hemp seed, chia, flax, or evening primrose. These omega-containing seeds and oils contain the essential nutrients EPA and DHA (long-chain essential fatty acids) found in fish oil. The key to supplementation is ensuring you are getting the proper EPA and DHA ratio. This ratio is essential to avoid potentially serious health problems. If you consume enough whole foods and vegetable oils, you are most likely getting enough omega-6 in your diet. It is then omega-3 that becomes important because it has the metabolites of EPA and DHA when taken in the right form.

Reputable manufacturers offer reliable supplements, but as always it comes down to reading and understanding the label lingo. Just remember to balance omega-3s with healthy omega-6 vegetable oils. A healthy diet along with topical beauty products made with essential fatty acids is the perfect combo for a naturally youthful and radiant complexion!

Mind/Body Beauty

Renew with Meditation and Relaxation!

Do you know that you can achieve beauty with daily stress relief? It's true! Meditation is an ancient technique used for thousands of years across cultures to reduce stress and quiet the mind. Meditation practices like yoga are getting a lot of attention and today scientists are finding that a daily meditation can provide many benefits including:

- Reducing daily stress levels
- Increasing energy
- Helping you sleep better
- Improving circulation
- Supporting a healthy immune system
- Improving your mood

All of these benefits also result in improvements in appearance and outlook. Those who meditate can reduce their stress levels, obtain more restful sleep, look and feel better, and be healthier overall. They also benefit from fewer lines and wrinkles, less acne, and a healthy glow that's only possible by maintaining mind/body balance. Meditation provides a simple solution to lasting beauty and wellness.

Meditation not only supports good physical health, but also promotes a strong mind/body connection and spiritual growth. Who isn't more vibrant, energized, and beautiful when she's happy? Consider how a physically beautiful person looks when she's angry or mean-spirited. Not so pretty, right? What's on the inside shows on the outside. Whether it's a poor diet or a mind full of negativity, your appearance reveals what's going on inside.

Meditation benefits can be achieved in as little as *15 minutes a day*! That's great news for us busy, stressed-out folks managing a multitude of tasks on a daily basis. Try a quick 15-minute morning meditation and simply take those quiet moments when you first wake to begin your practice. It's always easier to maintain a clear mind rather than try to attain one amidst a hectic environment.

Breathe for Beauty

When you are under stress, your body produces large amounts of the stress hormone cortisol. Normal levels of cortisol are healthy and can boost your everyday performance. Unfortunately, given today's hectic lifestyle, chances are that your cortisol levels are constantly peaking. Excess cortisol can contribute to premature aging and have other negative effects like weight gain (especially around the mid-section).

Aside from inhibiting the production of cortisol, a meditation with deep breathing practice can also increase the melatonin production in your body. Unlike cortisol, melatonin can slow down the effects of aging.

Melatonin is a hormone that is usually associated with sleep. During bedtime, your melatonin level increases, making you feel sluggish and sleepy. When you wake up in the morning, your exposure to sunlight causes your melatonin levels to go down. But sleeping is not the only way to boost your melatonin levels.

Research has shown that breathing deeply on a regular basis can help restore your body's melatonin to a healthy level. You can do this via meditation or just incorporate deep breathing into your daily work breaks.

If this is your first time to try meditation and deep breathing, then you are probably uncertain as to how you should proceed. Try these tips to get started.

Tips for Meditation and Deep Breathing

Find a quiet place. Naturally, the first thing you need to do is look for a place in your home (or outdoors) where you won't be easily distracted by any noise or activities.

Focus on your breathing. Concentrating on your breathing is the simplest way to begin a meditation practice. Focus on the path your breath takes. Breathe in through the nose and out through the mouth.

Calmly clear your mind of all thoughts. When you find yourself getting distracted with thoughts, don't panic or feel frustrated. Let the thoughts come and go, and then gradually return to your breathing.

Keep practicing. Practice these techniques on a daily basis, and you will eventually master them and reap the rewards!

Bubbles or Not, Baths Are Fun – Rubber Ducky, You're the One!

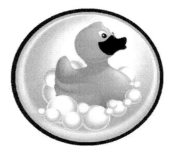

Another wonderful form of relaxation that has been used since ancient times is a bath. Bathing is an effective tool to remove stress, detoxify, and rejuvenate your senses. Gone are the days when bathing was simply for hygienic purposes. Nowadays, bathing is used for its healing and therapeutic effects as well.

Herbs, essential oils, and Dead Sea salts are some of the common additives used to make a bath experience truly soothing, therapeutic and indulgent. Meditation and bathing compliment one another because both alleviate a tired body and remove the clutters of the mind, bringing a sense of peace.

While meditation and bathing may not be conventional "beauty" treatments, when you add them to a lifestyle regimen that includes eating well, staying properly hydrated, using non-toxic products, and getting regular exercise, you'll see that both are important parts of a holistic lifestyle that will benefit your entire body, including your appearance.

Get started now, it's never too late!

Yoga for Youth

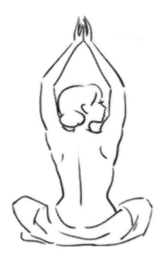

We all realize fitness activities are a good thing for our bodies, but did you know that fitness routines such as yoga improve your skin and overall beauty as well as your state of mind? Since most people's stress levels are often high, yoga is a great way to unwind and reap the benefits. Yoga maximizes flexibility to help avoid strains and pain and also improves circulation, which helps to minimize stress. Certain postures, or poses, called "Asanas," also bring blood to your face, which can reduce wrinkling. Some inverted postures offer improved circulation to the facial area, minimizing puffy eyes and dark circles, detoxifying, improving collagen production, and contributing to a radiant glow.

The reduced level of stress yoga practitioners experience is a better anti-aging remedy than any cream or potion. Also, the increased oxygenation of your blood from deep breathing done during yoga, as well as the increased circulation overall, helps remove toxins, thus improving skin tone and texture.

Ever Heard of Hot Yoga?

This yoga practice uses similar positions as Hatha Yoga but the room is heated up to help your muscles stretch better. It encourages a sweat to flush toxins out of your body naturally and improve the health of your skin. Hot yoga is a great way to rid your body (and your skin) of toxins, but make sure you don't get dehydrated, as that can be counterproductive for the skin and also risky for those with certain health conditions. So hydrate often!

New to Yoga?

A great way to observe these postures is by a simple internet search. Here are 3 simple Asanas to get you started:

1. Child's Pose (Balasana)

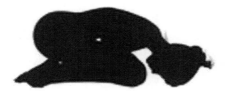

This is an ideal pose for anyone. Simply concentrate on your breathing and relax in this gentle forward position. First come to a seated position with your calves and feet tucked underneath your sitz bones (your bottom). Now, with a flat back reach gently forward with your belly resting between your open hips and legs. As you reach forward, rest your forearms and third eye (the imaginary eye in the center of your forehead between your eyes) onto your mat, and breathe gently. You may also rest your arms and hands along the outside of your legs with your palms up should this be more comfortable for you.

Child's Pose is a pose you can come to anytime in your practice, and it's also an excellent meditative pose that will bring peace to your entire day, and radiance to your skin!

2. Downward-Facing Dog (Svanasana)

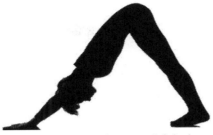

This great posture gently stretches the entire body while increasing the blood flow to your face, neck, and body, promoting a healthy, youthful glow.

Begin by coming onto all fours. If you'd like, you can do a few cat/cow poses. To do them, simply breathe in and arch your back pressing into your hands and out through your heels – then breathe out, releasing your breath while raising your head, heart and bottom, and dip your belly toward the ground.

With a flat back, on all fours press your hands and toes into the mat and raise your sitz bones to the sky. Your head will come naturally between your arms, but don't lock your elbows. And always remember to spread your fingers wide in order to distribute your weight evenly throughout your hands.

If you can flatten your feet comfortably go ahead, otherwise, bend your knees as needed, and breathe. Remember to inhale and exhale evenly throughout your yoga practice no matter what the pose. Downward-Facing Dog, like Child's Pose is another restful pose to return to any time in your practice to focus on your breath and regain your center.

3. **Standing Forward Bend (Uttanasana)**

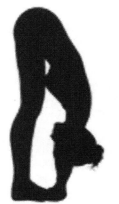

Your body is inverted when doing the Uttanasana/Standing Forward Bend position, which increases blood circulation and flow to your brain while you stretch your entire body, releasing toxins and contributing to enhanced collagen formation for more radiant skin.

Uttanasana is generally part of a sun salutation that also incorporates Downward-Facing Dog. Most begin Uttanasana from a standing position, with a straight back and arms extending out from the shoulders. Then fall gently forward on the next exhalation. If you can, keep your legs straight; if not, bend your knees gently and fold your hands behind your calves, or you can reach your fingertips to the floor beside or behind your heels, your head hanging gently from your shoulders. Breathe here for a few breaths, gently reaching toward the ground with the crown of your head and lengthening through your spine. Come back to standing on an inhalation by placing your hands onto your hips and gently rising back to a full standing position.

You will need to be able to move freely, so slip into comfy workout gear, slick on some toxin-free skincare products, and get ready to look and feel better! Exercise, in general, can increase circulation, prevent health issues, and improve skin tone. You may also consider cardiovascular exercise and weight training. Just be careful and always seek medical advice prior to starting any new activities.

No Bull -- Get Your Beauty Sleep!

Without a doubt, the importance of sleep is oftentimes undermined. Yet many people still prefer to stay up late or simply suffer from insomnia due to stress and other factors.

Your overall health plays an important part in the aging process. Most people do a lot of things that contribute to stress such as working too many hours, maintaining schedules that are unrealistic, keeping up with kids, a hectic lifestyle, and any number of other factors. In order for the body to function at its optimum level it is necessary to get adequate rest. A good night's sleep is the best way to preserve your youth and have a clear mind for all of those important daily activities.

You may be wondering, "But I'm so busy, so what if I don't get enough sleep?" Here's what can happen as a result of sleep deprivation:

Immune System Deterioration

Your immune system is very complex. Made up of many types of cells and proteins, it's responsible for keeping foreign infectious agents such as common cold or flu viruses free from our body. Your cells regenerate, along with important hormones as you sleep, and if you are always lacking sleep, your body's ability to respond against bacterial and viral infection decreases. A healthy immune system is essential for beautiful, clear, and vibrant skin and hair. Poor quality sleep can also lead to rashes and skin disorders.

Memory Impairment

A good night's sleep has the capacity to trigger changes in the brain that compromise your memory, mood, and so much more. In the past, Sigmund Freud suspected that what a person learned during the day is rehearsed in their dreams and that this process leads to the formation of memories. Recent evidence shows that memory is stabilized and enhanced as a person sleeps and that, during that time, the body produces hormones and chemicals involved in the regulation of everything from memory and mood to weight.

Physical Fatigue

Lack of sleep means that your performance during physical and mental tasks can become inadequate. If you lack sleep, you may feel lightheaded, dizzy, confused, and experience brain fog. No matter how much you eat, you may still feel hungry, which can also lead to unwanted weight gain. Adrenal fatigue may also set in, contributing to additional symptoms and weight problems.[32]

In summary, sleep deprivation can lead to all kinds of health problems, the worst of which include diseases and premature aging. That's right, lack of sleep can even accelerate the aging process!

But never fear, here are some things you can do to keep your skin healthy, youthful, and radiant:

- Sleep on a 400-thread count or higher pillowcase. These are softer and less harsh, resulting in less wrinkling of your skin due to face positioning during the sleep cycle. Try to sleep on your back and avoid pressing your face on one side, as this can actually lead to permanent creasing/wrinkles on the face.

- Cleanse your skin thoroughly to remove makeup and environmental impurities that may contribute to free radical damage. Follow with high-quality creams and oils to protect and nourish your skin during the precious sleep cycle. Skin cells regenerate at night, which is yet another reason adequate sleep and quality nourishing products are essential for lasting beauty.

- Try melatonin or a calming herbal tea like chamomile or valerian root if you have a difficult time falling asleep. Dried lavender blooms under your pillow can also help ease mental and/or physical tension before bedtime.

- Remove the electronics from your life after a certain time every night. These devices are mentally stimulating and can cause stress, so turn it all off at the same time every night. This can help get your body into a rhythm, so it knows when it's time for bed. Light should not be present during the sleep cycle, so remove brightly lit clocks or phones from the room as well.

- Try to sleep a full 6-9 hours whenever possible. Get an extra 30 minutes of rest by going to bed earlier or taking daily "power" naps. You will notice the difference in how you look and feel.

- Deep relaxing breaths are also useful along with a mantra such as "Om" repeated over and over slowly as you gently fall into slumber. Ommmmm....

Finale:
Top Ten No Bull Beauty Tips!

Healthy Holistic Habits

Here are the top 10 natural beauty and holistic living tips and tricks that make a No Bull Lifestyle easy! Not only will you achieve amazing beauty, but the planet will benefit too!

1. Incorporate More Fruits and Veggies into Your Diet

Eat at least one veggie-filled salad every day, and enjoy a special drink like the No Bull Beauty Smoothie as your new breakfast! It's scientifically proven that the more raw organic, nutrient-rich foods you eat, the more your body can take advantage of all the benefits these foods offer which will result in an overall healthier body – including more nourished skin and hair.

2. Exercise Regularly

Feeling down? Then get moving! Whether you enjoy gardening, hiking, walking the dog, kayaking, yoga, swimming, or just goofing around with the kids in the yard...just move. Exercise increases circulation and is essential for healthy skin and a healthier you! And when you exercise outside, your mood is even further elevated.

3. Get Plenty of Rest

One of the most important things you can do for your skin is getting a great night's sleep. Collagen production increases during the precious sleep cycle, thus firming the skin and preventing water loss. Growth hormones peak during sleep, initiating cellular repair and tissue healing. The ideal amount of sleep ranges from 6-9 hours of uninterrupted sleep per night. When you sleep well, the products you use may actually work more effectively, so it's a good idea to get plenty of rest.

4. Limit or Avoid Meat, Dairy, and Processed Foods

The more you avoid meat, dairy, processed foods, GMOs, and artificial "everything" the better the chances of improving your health and beauty, including reducing hormonal acne challenges, cholesterol, insulin, and more! Decreasing the amount of unhealthy foods you eat can make a big difference in the appearance of your skin, hair and overall wellness.

5. Seek Nutrient-Rich Ingredients

Utilize naturally-sourced ingredients from teas, plants, nuts, and berries that offer antioxidants, nutrients, and omega fatty acids. You'll find that these natural ingredients offer many more benefits for your skin and are easily absorbed and utilized by your body, when compared to their chemically derived counterparts. Plus, your skin absorbs *everything,* so consider that when you're reading ingredient lists.

6. Don't Worry Be Happy

A positive outlook means less stress and increased inner peace, which equates to a healthy glow. Seems so simple doesn't it? And it's true. It works, and it feels better! Smiling also releases endorphins (hormones that automatically reduce stress) and generates a positive feeling. Smiling is contagious, plus it takes less muscles to smile than it does to frown. When you are in a bad mood, try smiling (or even laughing) to improve your mood. Smile often, laugh a lot, worry less, enjoy life...happiness makes you more beautiful, naturally.

7. Avoid Synthetic Ingredients

Synthetics are in many different personal care and beauty products. Natural (when truly natural, of course) is better, and this goes for fragrances and air fresheners too, which contain icky phthalates and hormone disruptors. Toxic ingredients are harmful to your pets and the planet too, so toss them all today!

8. Use Toxin-Free Cleaning Products

What do cleaning products have to do with natural beauty? A lot! When you clean, your skin is exposed to the mist and chemicals of the products you're using. Choose or make your own natural products to protect your skin, your kids, your pets, and the planet!

9. Breathe Deeply

Deep breathing offers enhanced circulation and minimizes stress. Incorporating deep breathing exercises a few times a week will revive your skin, energy, and glow. Add in gentle stretching or yoga for a dynamic duo!

10. Meditate for Inner and Outer Beauty

Including meditation in your daily routine will not provide instant natural beauty benefits, but your entire mind, body and soul will thank you. Feeling like you can't fit one more thing into your hectic day? Even if you only meditate for just 15 minutes a day, you'll reap the rewards!

While adopting all ten of the No Bull Holistic Beauty Tips is ideal, following even just one of these tips can help reduce toxins both in your own body as well as in the Earth. Start today, and make a difference as early as tomorrow!

*And don't forget...*if you don't have a pet, consider one! With so many animals in need, it's easy to rescue one and do yourself as much good as the animal. Research has shown that pets can help decrease blood pressure, maintain healthy cholesterol levels, and reduce symptoms of depression and loneliness! Pets can bring so much happiness into your home, benefit your health, and make you smile. And when you smile more, you are naturally prettier! A pet also increases your opportunity for socialization and exercise. Love = natural beauty.

Namaste

So, did I cut through the crap enough for you? Stay alert and informed as new Bull is born every day. We can make an effort to "green it" together! It's never too late.

Join the No Bull mailing list and visit the No Bull Beauty Blog to stay up-to-date with the latest Bull, and learn more about living a non-toxic lifestyle. Please leave your comments, questions, concerns and info. I would love to hear from you!

If you would like to schedule a consultation, or to learn more about my non-toxic skincare formulations, visit: **www.NoBullBeauty.com** or **www.SevaniBeauty.com.**

"Truth never damages a cause that is just."
– Mahatma Gandhi

ABOUT THE AUTHOR

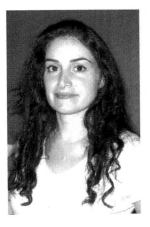

Sheryl Lynn Gibbs, Holistic Aesthetician, Cosmetologist, and founder of the No Bull Beauty Method, grew up battling allergies to processed foods and common ingredients found in modern body care creams, lotions, and cosmetics.

For the past 25 years, she has customized botanical skin treatments for a myriad of grateful clients. Currently a formulator of Sevani Botanica Skincare, she's not just an experienced Holistic Aesthetician, she's also an alchemist, who creates modern-day formulations to advance the skin care industry.

Also an experienced cosmetologist, she's a mad scientist of sorts with a vast knowledge of all things beauty. Her mission is to share this knowledge with not only her clients, but anyone interested to know how to nurture their health and maintain natural beauty. Sheryl can help you uncover all of the crap out there, so you can see what natural beauty really feels like, making her a refreshing presence in this world of toxins, chemicals, and pollutants.

Sheryl resides with her husband and 4 kitties: Lamont, Laverne, Gertrude, and Blanche, and whatever other fosters find their way into their hearts and homes. She is also a vigorous advocate for animals, of all kinds and the diverse and beautiful planet.

REFERENCES

1. Environmental Working Group. "Impurities of Concern in Personal Care Products." EWG'S Skin Deep Cosmetics Database. *February 2007.* (http://www.ewg.org/skindeep/2007/02/04/impurities-of-concern-in-personal-care-products/)

2. National Research Council. "Toxicity Testing." Washington, D.C.: National Academy Press, 1984. (http://www.nap.edu/openbook.php?isbn=0309034337)

3. EPA's Computational Toxicology Research. "EPA Research Progress Report." (2012). (http://www.epa.gov/ncct/)

4. A, Aljarrah, PD, Darbre. "Concentrations of Parabens in Human Breast Tumors." *JAT: Journal of Applied Toxicology.* 2004 Jan-Feb;24(1):5-13. *J Appl Toxicol.* July 2010; 29 (4). (http://www.ncbi.nlm.nih.gov/pubmed/14745841)

5. Exog Dermatol 2004;3:19-25 (DOI:10.1159/000084139) "A comparison Study of Nonanoic Acid and Sodium Lauryl Sulfate in Skin Irritation." (http://www.karger.com/Article/FullText/84139)

6. Report by the Committee on Science and Technology. U.S. House of Representatives. [Report 99-827] Sept. 16, 1986.

7. U.S. EPA Hazard Summary. "Hydroquinone." 2010. (http://www.epa.gov/ttnatw01/hlthef/hydroqui.html)

8. Material Safety Data Sheet. "Benzoyl peroxide MSDS." 2012.(http://www.sciencelab.com/msds.php?msdsId=9923 063)

9. Fox, Maggie. "Common Disinfectant Could Breed Superbugs." *Encoura*. (http://www.encoura.com/products/media/common.htm)

10. American Cancer Society. "Skin Cancer Prevention and Early Detection." 2012. (http://www.cancer.org/acs/groups/cid/documents/webcont ent/003184-pdf.pdf)

11. Environmental Working Group. "CDC: Americans Carry Body Burden of Toxic Sunscreen Chemical." 2008. (http://www.ewg.org/research/cdc-americans-carry-body-burden-toxic-sunscreen-chemical)

12. Environmental Working Group. "The Trouble With Sunscreen Chemicals." 2013. Web. http://www.ewg.org/2013sunscreen/the-trouble-with-sunscreen-chemicals/

13. A) "Are 'Spray-On'Tans Safe? Experts Raise Questions as Industry Puts Out Warning." 2012. (http://abcnews.go.com/Health/safety-popular-spray-tans-question-protected/story?id=16542918#.UaVP5pVg14G)

B) "Dihydroxyacetone, the active browning ingredient in sunless tanning lotions, induces DNA damage, cell-cycle block and apoptosis in cultured HaCaT keratinocytes." Res. 2004 June 13;560(2);173-86 (http://www.ncbi.nlm.nih.gov/pubmed/15157655)

14. ATSDR, Agency for Toxic Substances and Disease Registry. "ToxFAQ's for Aluminum." 2008. (http://www.atsdr.cdc.gov/toxfaqs/tf.asp?id=190&tid=34)

15. RC, Hamdy. "Aluminum Toxicity and Alzheimer's Disease. Is There a Connection?" College of Medicine, East Tennessee State University, Johnson City. Postgrad Med. 1990 Oct;88(5):239-40. (http://www.ncbi.nlm.nih.gov/pubmed/2216983)

16. S, Brenner. "Aluminum May Mediate Alzheimer's Disease Through Liver Toxicity, with Aberrant Hepatic Synthesis of Ceruloplasmin and ATPase7B, the Resultant Excess Free Copper Causing Brain Oxidation, Beta-Amyloid Aggregation and Alzheimer Disease." Med Hypotheses. 2013 Mar;80(3):326-7. (http://www.ncbi.nlm.nih.gov/pubmed/23261179)

17. Harlow BL, Cramer DW. "Perineal exposure to talc and ovarian cancer risk." Obstetrics & Gynecology, 80: 19-26, 1992. (http://www.ncbi.nlm.nih.gov/pubmed/1603491)

18. Department of Health and Human Services, U.S. Food and Drug Administration. "Mercury Poisoning Linked to Skin Products." 2013.

(http://www.fda.gov/ForConsumers/ConsumerUpdates/uc
m294849.htm)

19. Hemphill, Meghan. "We Eat 7 Pounds of Lipstick."
    Huffington Post. 2009.
    (http://www.huffingtonpost.com/meg-hemphill/we-eat-7-
    pounds-of-lipsti_b_391323.html)

20. Department of Health and Human Services, U.S. Food and
    Drug Administration. "Lipstick and Lead: Questions and
    Answers."
    (http://www.fda.gov/cosmetics/productandingredientsafety
    /productinformation/ucm137224.htm)

21. California Department of Public Health. "California
    Childhood Lead Poisoning Prevention Branch: Children at
    Risk." 2013.
    (http://www.cdph.ca.gov/healthinfo/discond/Pages/CLPPB
    ChildrenATRisk.aspx)

22. USDA National Organic Program. "Testing for Prohibited
    Substances in USDA Organic Products." 2013.
    (http://www.ams.usda.gov/AMSv1.0/getfile?dDocName=
    STELPRDC5101208)

23. Hennessey, Rachel. "GMO Food Debate in the National
    Spotlight." 2012.
    (http://www.forbes.com/sites/rachelhennessey/2012/11/03/
    gmo-food-debate-in-the-national-spotlight/)

24. Department of Health and Human Services, U.S. Food and Drug Administration. "Questions & Answers on Food from Genetically Engineered Plants." 2013. (http://www.fda.gov/Food/FoodScienceResearch/Biotechnology/ucm346030.htm)

25. EWG's Skin Deep Sunscreens 2012. "The Problem With Vitamin A. Sunscreens." 2012. (http://www.ewg.org/2012sunscreen/sunscreens-exposed/the-problem-with-vitamin-a/)

26. Hartman RE, Shah A. "Pomegranate juice decreases amyloid load and improves behavior in a mouse model of Alzheimer's disease." Neurobiology of Diseases. 2006 Dec;24(3):506-15. Epub 2006 Sep 28. (http://www.ncbi.nlm.nih.gov/pubmed/17010630)

27. Cappel M, Mauger D. "Correlation Between Serum Levels of Insulin-Like Growth Factor 1, Dehydroepiandrosterone Sulfate, and Dihydrotestosterone and Acne Lesion Counts in Adult Women." Archives of Dermatology. 2005.Mar;141(3):333-8. (http://www.ncbi.nlm.nih.gov/pubmed/15781674)

28. Gardner, Christopher D., Coulston, Ann. "The Effect of a Plant-Based Diet on Plasma Lipids in Hypercholesterolemic Adults A Randomized Trial." Annals of Internal Medicine. 2005; 142:725-733. (http://nutrition.stanford.edu/documents/Plant_based.pdf)

29. Adisen, Esra, Kaymak Yesim. "Zinc Levels in Patients with Acne Vulgaris." Journal of the Turkish Academy of Dermatology. 2007; 1 (3): 71302a. (http://www.jtad.org/2007/3/jtad71302a.pdf)

30. Youseff, Dima A. Miller. "Antimicrobial Implications of Vitamin D." Dermatoendocrinol. 2001; Oct-Dec; 3(4):220-229. (http://www.ncbi.nlm.nih.gov/pmc/articles/PMC3256336/)

31. Pogge E. "Vitamin D and Alzheimer's Disease: Is There a Link?" The Consultant Pharmacist. (2010 Jul, 25 (7) 440-50). (http://www.ncbi.nlm.nih.gov/pubmed/20601349)

32. WebMD. "Sleep Deprivation and Memory Loss. WebMd. Web." 2013. (http://www.webmd.com/sleep-disorders/sleep-deprivation-effects-on-memory)

Made in the USA
Lexington, KY
15 May 2014